PRINCIPLES OF HEALTHY LIVING

Why We Get Sick---Decoding the Underlying Epidemic Fueling Numerous Chronic Diseases and Strategies for Resilience

By

Calvin M. Duncan

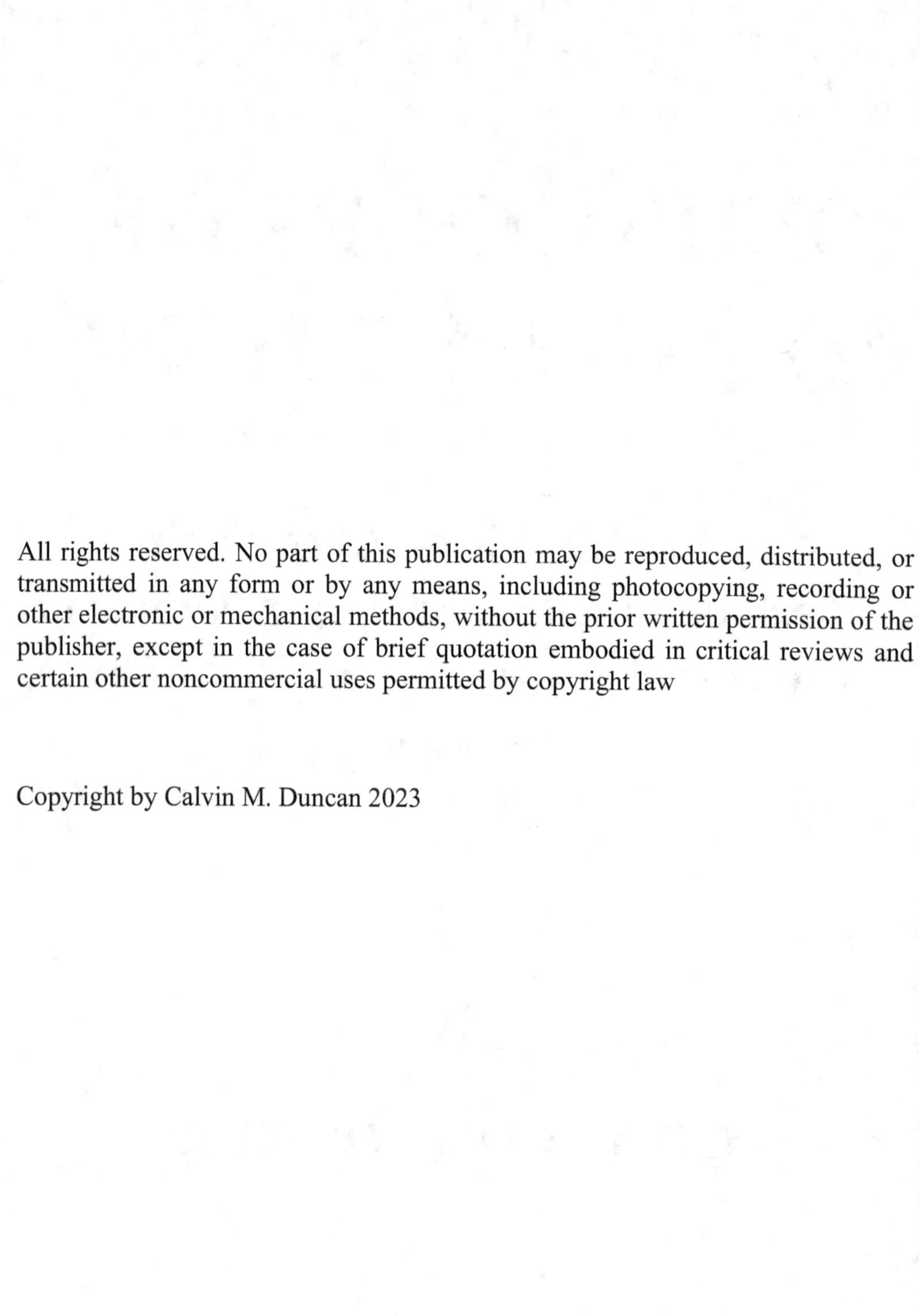

TABLE OF CONTENTS

Introduction

Chapter 1: The Roots of Illness

- Genetic Predispositions

- Environmental Triggers

- Lifestyle Factors

Chapter 2: The Inflammatory Connection

- Inflammation's Role in Chronic Disease

- Identifying and Addressing Chronic Inflammatory Processes

Chapter 3: The Microbial Symphony

- Gut Microbiota and Health

- Microbial Dysbiosis in Chronic Conditions

Chapter 4: Navigating the Immune System

- Immune Dysfunction and Chronic Diseases

- Strategies for Modulating the Immune Response

Chapter 5: The Impact of Modern Living

- Technological Advances and Health Consequences

- Urbanization, Stress, and Their Toll on Well-being

Chapter 6: Dietary Patterns and Disease

- The Role of Nutrition in Chronic Conditions

- Crafting a Healing Diet

Chapter 7: Beyond Pharmaceuticals

- Integrative Approaches to Treatment

- Holistic Healing Modalities

Chapter 8: Prevention Strategies

- Lifestyle Modifications for Disease Prevention

- Public Health Initiatives

Chapter 9: Building Resilience

- Strengthening the Body's Natural Defenses

- Cultivating Mental and Emotional Well-being

Chapter 10: The Future of Health

- Innovations in Medicine and Wellness

- A Roadmap for a Healthier Society

Conclusion

- Empowering Individuals for Lasting Health

- Real-life Examples of Disease Reversal and Prevention

INTRODUCTION

Unveiling the Hidden Epidemic

In the quest to understand the complex interplay of factors contributing to the rise of chronic diseases, it becomes imperative to delve into the depths of the hidden epidemic that underlies these pervasive health challenges. Chronic diseases, ranging from cardiovascular issues to autoimmune disorders, have become increasingly prevalent in modern society. This epidemic is not always apparent at first glance, as it operates beneath the surface, weaving its intricate web of causative factors. Unveiling this hidden epidemic requires a comprehensive exploration of the various elements that converge to fuel the fire of chronic illness.

At the core of this hidden epidemic are intricate connections between genetics, environment, and lifestyle. The human genome, a masterpiece of biological complexity, holds clues to our susceptibility to certain diseases. Genetic predispositions can create a foundation upon which environmental triggers and lifestyle choices exert their influence. Understanding the nuances of these interactions is crucial for unraveling the mystery behind the surge in chronic conditions.

Environmental factors play a pivotal role in the unfolding narrative of chronic diseases. The modern world is rife with pollutants, toxins, and stressors that assail the body's delicate equilibrium. From air and water quality to the chemicals found in everyday products, our environment has undergone significant changes over the years. Uncovering how these environmental factors contribute to the development and progression of chronic diseases is paramount in designing effective prevention and intervention strategies.

Lifestyle choices, too, are integral to the equation. Diet, exercise, sleep patterns, and stress management all play pivotal roles in shaping our health outcomes. The sedentary nature of modern living, coupled with diets high in processed foods, has created a breeding ground for chronic inflammation—a hallmark of many chronic diseases. Delving into the lifestyle factors that promote or undermine health is essential for formulating actionable plans to mitigate the impact of this hidden epidemic.

Chronic inflammation emerges as a central player in the orchestration of chronic diseases. It is the body's response to a variety of stimuli, including infections, environmental toxins, and poor dietary choices. While acute inflammation is a protective response, chronic inflammation can become a destructive force, contributing to the development and progression of conditions such as diabetes, heart disease, and autoimmune disorders. Unraveling the intricacies of the inflammatory response is key to understanding how it becomes dysregulated in the context of chronic diseases.

The microbiome, an ecosystem of trillions of microbes residing in the human body, adds another layer to the hidden epidemic. The gut microbiota, in particular, has emerged as a critical player in

health and disease. Imbalances in the microbial community within the gut have been linked to a myriad of health issues, from gastrointestinal disorders to mental health conditions. Exploring the dynamic relationship between the microbiome and chronic diseases provides valuable insights into potential therapeutic interventions and preventive measures.

As we navigate the terrain of chronic diseases, the immune system emerges as a sentinel standing guard against threats to our well-being. However, in the context of chronic conditions, the immune system can become dysregulated, either overactive or underactive. Understanding the delicate balance required for optimal immune function is crucial for developing targeted interventions to prevent and treat chronic diseases.

Modern living, characterized by technological advances and urbanization, has brought about profound changes in our daily lives. While these changes have undoubtedly improved certain aspects of our existence, they have also introduced new challenges to our health. From increased screen time and sedentary behavior to the stressors of city life, the impact of modern living on our health cannot be overlooked. Unraveling the ways in which these changes influence chronic disease patterns provides valuable insights into crafting holistic approaches to health promotion.

Diet, a cornerstone of health, is a multifaceted aspect of the hidden epidemic. The modern diet, often characterized by high levels of processed foods, sugars, and unhealthy fats, contributes significantly to the development of chronic diseases. Conversely, a diet rich in nutrients, antioxidants, and anti-inflammatory compounds can serve as a powerful tool for prevention and intervention. Examining the intricate relationship between dietary patterns and chronic diseases is essential for developing evidence-based nutritional strategies.

Beyond the traditional pharmaceutical model, integrative approaches to treatment offer a promising avenue for addressing the hidden epidemic of chronic diseases. Incorporating complementary therapies, lifestyle modifications, and mind-body practices into conventional medical care can enhance overall well-being and improve treatment outcomes. Exploring the synergy between conventional and alternative modalities provides a holistic framework for managing chronic conditions.

As we contemplate prevention strategies, the importance of lifestyle modifications comes to the forefront. Small changes in daily habits, such as regular exercise, stress management techniques, and a nutrient-dense diet, can have profound effects on health outcomes. Public health initiatives aimed at promoting these lifestyle modifications on a broader scale can contribute to stemming the tide of the hidden epidemic.

Building resilience becomes a paramount consideration in the face of the hidden epidemic. Strengthening the body's natural defenses and fostering mental and emotional well-being are integral components of resilience. Exploring the strategies and practices that contribute to resilience equips individuals with the tools needed to navigate the challenges presented by chronic diseases.

Real-life case studies serve as poignant illustrations of the potential for disease reversal and prevention. Examining individuals who have successfully overcome chronic conditions provides

valuable insights into the factors and interventions that contribute to positive outcomes. These stories offer hope and inspiration to others facing similar health challenges.

Looking toward the future, innovations in medicine and wellness hold the promise of transformative change. From personalized medicine based on genetic profiles to advancements in preventive strategies, the landscape of healthcare is evolving. A roadmap for a healthier society involves embracing these innovations while also advocating for systemic changes that prioritize health promotion and disease prevention.

In conclusion, unveiling the hidden epidemic fueling chronic disease requires a multidimensional exploration of genetics, environment, lifestyle, inflammation, the microbiome, immune function, modern living, diet, and innovative approaches to treatment and prevention. By understanding the intricate web of factors contributing to chronic diseases, we can develop informed strategies to address this pervasive health challenge and pave the way for a healthier future.

The Landscape of Chronic Disease

Chronic diseases, once considered ailments of the elderly or a consequence of genetic predispositions, have become an alarming global phenomenon affecting individuals across age groups and backgrounds. As we survey the landscape of chronic disease, it becomes evident that this terrain is vast, complex, and continually evolving. Understanding the multifaceted nature of chronic diseases is crucial for both healthcare professionals and the general public, as it informs prevention strategies, treatment modalities, and the allocation of resources in the pursuit of better public health outcomes.

At the heart of the chronic disease landscape lies a staggering array of conditions, each with its unique characteristics, risk factors, and impacts on individuals and communities. From cardiovascular diseases like hypertension and coronary artery disease to metabolic disorders such as diabetes, and from autoimmune conditions like rheumatoid arthritis to neurodegenerative disorders like Alzheimer's, the scope of chronic diseases is far-reaching. This diversity underscores the challenge of addressing chronic diseases comprehensively and necessitates a nuanced approach tailored to the specificities of each condition.

The prevalence of chronic diseases has witnessed a remarkable surge in recent decades, prompting a shift in healthcare priorities worldwide. While infectious diseases have historically dominated public health concerns, the escalating burden of chronic conditions demands a paradigm shift in our approach to healthcare. This shift is not only in response to the increasing numbers of individuals affected but also to the substantial impact chronic diseases have on healthcare systems, economies, and overall societal well-being.

The demographic landscape contributes significantly to the prevalence of chronic diseases. Aging populations, a global phenomenon, are particularly susceptible to chronic conditions. The gradual wear and tear on the body's systems over time, coupled with a lifetime of exposures to various risk factors, contribute to the higher incidence of chronic diseases in older age. However, it is essential to recognize that chronic diseases are not exclusive to the elderly; an alarming rise in chronic conditions among younger populations has become a cause for concern.

The interplay between genetic predispositions and environmental factors shapes the trajectory of chronic diseases. While genetics lays the foundation for an individual's susceptibility to certain conditions, it is the environment that often triggers the onset or exacerbation of these diseases. Genetic factors alone do not account for the surge in chronic diseases; it is the interaction between genes and the environment that creates a fertile ground for these conditions to flourish.

The lifestyle choices individuals make further contribute to the landscape of chronic diseases. Diet, physical activity, sleep patterns, and stress management are all modifiable factors that play pivotal roles in health outcomes. The shift towards sedentary lifestyles, coupled with diets high in processed foods and sugars, has become a hallmark of the modern era. These lifestyle choices contribute to the rise of conditions such as obesity, type 2 diabetes, and cardiovascular diseases, shaping the landscape of chronic diseases in profound ways.

Inflammation, both acute and chronic, emerges as a common thread weaving through the landscape of chronic diseases. While acute inflammation is a natural and protective response to injuries or infections, chronic inflammation can become a driver of many chronic conditions. It is the silent force behind conditions like atherosclerosis, arthritis, and neurodegenerative disorders. Understanding the role of inflammation in the pathogenesis of chronic diseases provides a critical insight for developing targeted interventions.

The microbiome, a dynamic community of microorganisms inhabiting the human body, is a relatively recent addition to our understanding of the landscape of chronic diseases. The gut microbiota, in particular, plays a pivotal role in health and disease. Imbalances in the composition of the microbiome have been linked to conditions as diverse as inflammatory bowel disease, obesity, and mental health disorders. Exploring the intricate relationship between the microbiome and chronic diseases opens new avenues for therapeutic interventions and preventive strategies.

The immune system, tasked with defending the body against invaders, also occupies a central position in the landscape of chronic diseases. Dysregulation of the immune response can lead to autoimmune disorders, where the body mistakenly attacks its tissues, or contribute to chronic inflammatory conditions. Understanding the delicate balance required for optimal immune

function is crucial for unraveling the complexities of chronic diseases and developing immunomodulatory therapies.

Modern living, characterized by technological advancements and urbanization, has introduced novel challenges to health. Sedentary behavior, increased screen time, and the stressors of city life all contribute to the landscape of chronic diseases. These factors not only directly impact health but also influence lifestyle choices and access to healthcare, creating disparities that further complicate the management of chronic conditions.

Diet, a cornerstone of health, is a significant determinant of the chronic disease landscape. The modern diet, often characterized by convenience foods high in sugars, unhealthy fats, and additives, contributes to the rise of conditions like obesity, diabetes, and cardiovascular diseases. Conversely, a diet rich in fruits, vegetables, whole grains, and lean proteins can serve as a powerful preventive measure and therapeutic intervention for chronic diseases.

Beyond the conventional pharmaceutical model, integrative approaches to treatment offer a holistic perspective on managing chronic diseases. Incorporating complementary therapies, lifestyle modifications, and mind-body practices into conventional medical care can enhance overall well-being and improve treatment outcomes. The landscape of chronic diseases, with its complexity, demands a multifaceted and patient-centered approach to care.

Prevention strategies, the cornerstone of public health, play a pivotal role in shaping the landscape of chronic diseases. Efforts aimed at promoting healthy lifestyles, early detection of risk factors, and community-based interventions contribute to reducing the burden of chronic conditions. Public health initiatives that address social determinants of health, such as education, income, and access to healthcare, are integral to reshaping the landscape and fostering a culture of health.

Building resilience within individuals and communities becomes a crucial aspect of navigating the landscape of chronic diseases. Strengthening the body's natural defenses, fostering mental and emotional well-being, and creating supportive environments contribute to resilience. Individuals equipped with the tools to face the challenges posed by chronic diseases are better positioned to manage their conditions effectively and lead fulfilling lives.

Real-life case studies offer poignant narratives within the landscape of chronic diseases. Examining individuals who have successfully managed or overcome chronic conditions provides valuable insights into the factors and interventions that contribute to positive outcomes. These stories not only highlight the resilience of the human spirit but also serve as beacons of hope for others facing similar health challenges.

As we gaze into the future, the landscape of chronic diseases is marked by both challenges and opportunities. Innovations in medicine, technology, and public health hold the promise of transformative change. Personalized medicine, advancements in preventive strategies, and a growing emphasis on patient-centered care offer new avenues for reshaping the landscape and improving health outcomes.

In conclusion, the landscape of chronic diseases is a dynamic and multifaceted terrain shaped by genetics, environment, lifestyle, inflammation, the microbiome, immune function, modern living,

diet, and innovative approaches to treatment and prevention. Navigating this landscape requires a comprehensive understanding of the intricate web of factors that contribute to chronic diseases. By unraveling these complexities, we can develop informed strategies to address the challenges posed by chronic conditions and work towards building a healthier and more resilient future.

CHAPTER ONE

Genetic Predispositions of Chronic Illness

The human genome, a magnificent tapestry of over 20,000 genes, serves as the intricate blueprint for our biological existence. Within this vast genetic code lie not only the instructions for the color of our eyes and the shape of our noses but also the potential susceptibilities to various health conditions, including chronic illnesses. Genetic predispositions, the inherent genetic factors that influence an individual's likelihood of developing specific health conditions, play a pivotal role in shaping the landscape of chronic diseases.

Understanding genetic predispositions involves peering into the complex interplay between an individual's genetic makeup and the environmental factors that surround them. Genes provide the basic framework for our biological functions, but it is the interaction between these genes and the environment that determines whether certain predispositions will manifest as chronic diseases. Unraveling the mysteries of genetic predispositions requires delving into the fundamentals of genetics, exploring the mechanisms through which genes influence health, and deciphering the ways in which environmental factors modify these genetic predispositions.

At the heart of genetic predispositions is the concept of heritability, the degree to which genetic factors contribute to the variability of traits within a population. Some traits, like eye color, are highly heritable and are primarily determined by genetic factors. When it comes to chronic diseases, the interplay between genetics and environment becomes more intricate. Certain conditions, such as diabetes and cardiovascular diseases, have a significant heritable component, meaning that individuals with a family history of these conditions are at an increased risk.

The journey into the world of genetic predispositions begins with a fundamental exploration of the structure and function of DNA. Deoxyribonucleic acid, commonly known as DNA, is the molecular foundation of genetics. Comprising a double helix structure, DNA consists of nucleotide base pairs that encode the instructions for building and maintaining an organism. The sequence of these base pairs is unique to each individual and forms the basis of their genetic code.

Genes, the functional units within DNA, serve as the blueprint for the production of proteins, the building blocks of life. Proteins play diverse roles in the body, from catalyzing chemical reactions to providing structure to cells and tissues. The expression of genes, the process through which the information encoded in DNA is used to create proteins, is tightly regulated and influenced by both genetic and environmental factors.

Genetic variations, or polymorphisms, contribute to the diversity observed within the human population. These variations can occur at the level of a single nucleotide, known as single nucleotide polymorphisms (SNPs), or involve larger segments of DNA. The presence of specific

variations in certain genes can influence an individual's susceptibility to chronic diseases. While some variations may increase the risk of a particular condition, others may confer protective effects.

The concept of penetrance adds another layer of complexity to genetic predispositions. Penetrance refers to the proportion of individuals with a specific genetic variation who actually develop the associated trait or condition. Some genetic predispositions exhibit high penetrance, meaning that individuals with the genetic variation almost inevitably develop the condition. In contrast, low penetrance indicates that the genetic variation does not always result in the manifestation of the trait, highlighting the influence of other factors, such as the environment.

Identifying specific genes associated with chronic diseases is a crucial aspect of unraveling genetic predispositions. Genome-wide association studies (GWAS) have become instrumental in this endeavor, allowing researchers to scan the entire genome for genetic variations associated with particular conditions. These studies have revealed a multitude of genes linked to various chronic diseases, providing valuable insights into the genetic landscape of conditions such as diabetes, heart disease, and cancer.

The genetic basis of complex chronic diseases often involves the interaction of multiple genes, each contributing a small effect. This polygenic nature complicates the identification of specific genes responsible for a particular condition. Moreover, the genetic architecture of chronic diseases is often intertwined with environmental factors, making it challenging to disentangle the contributions of genes and the environment.

Family studies provide a tangible illustration of the heritability of chronic diseases. Observing patterns of disease occurrence within families allows researchers to estimate the genetic component of a particular condition. Families with a history of certain chronic diseases often exhibit a higher prevalence of these conditions among relatives, indicating a genetic predisposition. Twin studies, which compare the occurrence of diseases in identical and non-identical twins, further contribute to our understanding of the heritability of chronic diseases.

Genetic testing has emerged as a powerful tool for identifying specific genetic variations associated with chronic diseases. Advances in technology have made it increasingly feasible to sequence an individual's entire genome or focus on specific genes of interest. Genetic testing not only allows for the identification of known risk factors but also facilitates the discovery of novel genetic variations associated with chronic diseases. However, the ethical implications, potential psychological impact, and limitations of genetic testing warrant careful consideration.

While genetic predispositions undoubtedly influence the risk of chronic diseases, the environment plays a crucial role in modifying these genetic factors. The concept of gene-environment interaction recognizes that the expression of genetic predispositions is not predetermined but depends on the context of environmental exposures. Environmental factors, ranging from lifestyle choices and dietary habits to exposure to pollutants and stressors, can either amplify or mitigate the effects of genetic predispositions.

Epigenetics, the study of changes in gene expression that do not involve alterations to the underlying DNA sequence, provides a mechanistic understanding of how the environment influences genetic predispositions. Epigenetic modifications, such as DNA methylation and histone acetylation, can be influenced by environmental factors and serve as a molecular bridge between genes and the environment. These modifications can alter the accessibility of genes, influencing their expression and, consequently, the risk of chronic diseases.

The Developmental Origins of Health and Disease (DOHaD) hypothesis further underscores the impact of early-life exposures on genetic predispositions. This hypothesis posits that environmental influences during critical periods of development, such as fetal development and early childhood, can have lasting effects on health outcomes. Adverse environmental conditions during these sensitive periods can modify gene expression patterns, setting the stage for the later development of chronic diseases.

The intergenerational transmission of genetic predispositions adds another layer of complexity to the relationship between genes and chronic diseases. The experiences and exposures of one generation can influence the health outcomes of subsequent generations through mechanisms such as epigenetic inheritance. Understanding these transgenerational effects broadens our perspective on the long-term consequences of genetic predispositions and highlights the importance of a life-course approach to chronic disease prevention.

As we navigate the intricate landscape of genetic predispositions and chronic diseases, it is essential to acknowledge the role of genetic diversity within populations. Different populations may exhibit distinct genetic variations that influence their susceptibility to specific conditions. The field of pharmacogenomics, which examines how genetic variations impact an individual's response to medications, exemplifies the importance of considering genetic diversity in healthcare.

The translation of genetic discoveries into clinical practice represents a transformative frontier in the field of precision medicine. Tailoring medical interventions based on an individual's genetic profile holds the promise of more effective and personalized healthcare. Genetic information can guide treatment decisions, predict disease risk, and inform preventive strategies. However, the integration of genetics into clinical practice requires addressing challenges related to data interpretation, ethical considerations, and the need for robust evidence supporting the clinical utility of genetic information.

In conclusion, the genetic predispositions of chronic illness weave a complex tapestry that encompasses the blueprint of our health. Understanding the interplay between genetics and the environment, identifying specific genes associated with chronic diseases, and

 recognizing the impact of epigenetics and early-life exposures are integral to unraveling the mysteries of genetic predispositions. While genetic testing and precision medicine hold promise for personalized healthcare, a comprehensive approach that considers genetic diversity, gene-environment interactions, and the intergenerational transmission of genetic information is essential. As we delve deeper into the genetic foundations of chronic diseases, we move closer to a future where healthcare is not only tailored to the individual but also informed by a nuanced understanding of the intricate dance between genes and the environment.

Environmental Triggers of Chronic Diseases

The landscape of chronic diseases is not solely shaped by genetics; it is profoundly influenced by the environment in which individuals live, work, and play. Environmental triggers, encompassing a broad array of factors such as pollutants, lifestyle choices, and occupational exposures, play a pivotal role in the development and progression of chronic illnesses.

Unraveling the complex interplay between genetic predispositions and environmental triggers is essential for understanding the multifaceted origins of chronic diseases.

The modern world has witnessed unprecedented changes in the environment, driven by industrialization, urbanization, and technological advancements. While these changes have undoubtedly brought about improvements in many aspects of human life, they have also introduced new challenges to our health. Environmental triggers, both tangible and insidious, contribute to the rising tide of chronic diseases, affecting populations globally.

One of the most pervasive environmental triggers is air pollution. The air we breathe, once considered a source of life-sustaining oxygen, is increasingly tainted by pollutants emitted from vehicles, industrial facilities, and other human activities. Particulate matter, nitrogen dioxide, sulfur dioxide, and ozone are among the pollutants that can infiltrate the respiratory system, leading to a range of health issues. Long-term exposure to air pollution has been linked to respiratory conditions such as asthma and chronic obstructive pulmonary disease (COPD), as well as cardiovascular diseases and even certain cancers.

Water, a fundamental resource for life, is not immune to environmental contaminants. Industrial discharges, agricultural runoff, and inadequate wastewater treatment contribute to the contamination of water sources with chemicals, heavy metals, and pathogens. Contaminated water poses significant health risks, leading to waterborne diseases, gastrointestinal issues, and, in some cases, chronic conditions. The environmental impact on water quality is a silent contributor to the burden of chronic diseases, affecting communities that lack access to clean and safe water.

The food we consume, an essential aspect of daily life, is intricately linked to environmental triggers of chronic diseases. Modern agricultural practices, characterized by the use of pesticides, herbicides, and fertilizers, introduce chemical residues into the food chain. Additionally, the widespread availability of processed and convenience foods, often high in sugars, unhealthy fats, and additives, contributes to the rise of conditions such as obesity, diabetes, and cardiovascular diseases. Unraveling the environmental influences on the food we eat is essential for crafting strategies that promote healthier diets and mitigate the impact of dietary factors on chronic diseases.

Occupational exposures represent another facet of environmental triggers that can contribute to chronic diseases. Individuals working in certain industries may encounter hazardous substances, such as asbestos, heavy metals, and carcinogenic chemicals, as part of their job responsibilities. Prolonged exposure to these occupational hazards can lead to respiratory diseases, cancers, and

other chronic health conditions. Understanding the occupational determinants of chronic diseases is crucial for implementing workplace safety measures and protective policies.

Chemical exposures extend beyond the workplace to the products we use in our daily lives. The pervasive use of synthetic chemicals in household cleaners, personal care products, and plastics introduces a myriad of substances into our living environments. Some of these chemicals, such as endocrine-disrupting compounds, have been linked to hormonal imbalances, reproductive issues, and an increased risk of certain cancers. Unmasking the environmental triggers embedded in the products we interact with daily is essential for promoting safer alternatives and reducing the burden of chronic diseases.

Stress, often considered a psychological phenomenon, is also an environmental trigger with profound implications for health. The modern pace of life, marked by constant connectivity, information overload, and demanding work schedules, contributes to chronic stress levels. Chronic stress, in turn, can impact the immune system, cardiovascular function, and mental health. The environmental stressors of the modern world contribute to the rising prevalence of stress-related chronic conditions, including anxiety disorders, depression, and cardiovascular diseases.

The built environment, encompassing the design and layout of our communities, also plays a role in shaping the environmental triggers of chronic diseases. Urbanization, characterized by the concentration of populations in cities, has led to changes in lifestyle and exposure to environmental factors. Limited green spaces, air pollution, and sedentary lifestyles associated with urban living contribute to the burden of chronic diseases. Designing cities and communities that promote physical activity, access to nature, and environmental sustainability is essential for mitigating the impact of the built environment on health.

Climate change, a global environmental challenge, introduces a new dimension to the landscape of chronic diseases. Rising temperatures, extreme weather events, and shifts in precipitation patterns influence the spread of infectious diseases, the availability of food and water, and patterns of migration. These climate-related changes contribute to the emergence and reemergence of health threats, impacting vulnerable populations disproportionately. Addressing the health implications of climate change requires a holistic approach that considers the interconnectedness of environmental factors and their effects on chronic diseases.

The exposome, a concept encompassing the totality of environmental exposures throughout an individual's life, provides a framework for understanding the cumulative impact of environmental triggers on health. Unlike the genome, which remains relatively stable throughout life, the exposome is dynamic and influenced by a multitude of factors. Studying the exposome involves mapping the complex web of exposures individuals encounter, from air and water pollutants to dietary habits and lifestyle choices. The exposome concept underscores the need for comprehensive approaches to studying and addressing the environmental triggers of chronic diseases.

The developmental origins of health and disease (DOHaD) hypothesis, previously discussed in the context of genetic predispositions, also applies to environmental triggers. Exposures during critical periods of development, such as fetal development and early childhood, can have lasting effects on health outcomes. Environmental exposures during these sensitive periods can influence the risk of chronic diseases later in life, highlighting the importance of a life-course approach to understanding the impact of environmental triggers.

Unraveling the environmental triggers of chronic diseases requires interdisciplinary collaboration and innovative research methodologies. Epidemiological studies, which investigate the patterns and determinants of health in populations, play a crucial role in identifying associations between environmental exposures and chronic conditions. Biomonitoring, the measurement of environmental chemicals in biological samples, provides a direct assessment of an individual's exposure and allows for the identification of potential links to health outcomes.

Advances in technology, particularly in the field of environmental monitoring, offer new opportunities for understanding the environmental triggers of chronic diseases. Remote sensing, sensor networks, and big data analytics enable real-time monitoring of air and water quality, providing valuable insights into the dynamic nature of environmental exposures. Integrating these technological tools with traditional research approaches enhances our ability to identify, assess, and mitigate the impact of environmental triggers on health.

Public health interventions aimed at addressing environmental triggers of chronic diseases require a multifaceted approach. Regulation and policy measures can play a crucial role in reducing exposures to environmental pollutants and promoting healthier living environments. Advocacy for sustainable urban planning, clean energy initiatives, and waste reduction efforts contributes to broader environmental and health goals. Additionally, community-based interventions that empower individuals to make informed choices about their living environments and lifestyle habits are essential for promoting health at the grassroots level.

Environmental justice, a concept emphasizing the fair distribution of environmental benefits and burdens, is integral to addressing the environmental triggers of chronic diseases. Vulnerable populations, including low-income communities and minority groups, often bear a disproportionate burden of environmental exposures and the associated health risks. A commitment to environmental justice involves advocating for policies that reduce environmental health disparities and ensure equitable access to clean air, water, and living environments.

As we confront the environmental triggers of chronic diseases, it is essential to adopt a global perspective. Environmental challenges, such as air and water pollution, climate change, and exposure to hazardous substances, transcend national borders. Collaborative efforts at the international level are necessary to address these challenges comprehensively and implement solutions that promote planetary health. Global initiatives focused on sustainability, environmental protection, and public health contribute to a collective effort to mitigate the impact of environmental triggers on chronic diseases.

In conclusion, the environmental triggers of chronic diseases represent a complex web of factors that influence health outcomes on a global scale. From air and water pollution to occupational exposures, lifestyle choices, and climate change, the environmental landscape is vast and dynamic. Understanding the intricate interplay between genetic predispositions and environmental triggers is essential for unraveling the origins of chronic diseases and developing effective strategies for

prevention and intervention. As we navigate the challenges posed by environmental triggers, a commitment to environmental sustainability, justice, and global collaboration is paramount for creating a healthier and more resilient world.

Lifestyle Factors and Chronic Illness

In the complex tapestry of chronic illnesses, lifestyle factors emerge as critical threads that weave their influence on health outcomes. The choices individuals make in their daily lives, from dietary habits and physical activity levels to sleep patterns and stress management, play a profound role in shaping the risk and progression of chronic diseases. Understanding the intricate interplay between lifestyle factors and chronic illnesses is essential for developing effective prevention strategies and empowering individuals to take control of their health.

Diet, a cornerstone of lifestyle, stands as one of the most influential factors in the development and management of chronic illnesses. The modern era has witnessed significant shifts in dietary patterns, with an increasing reliance on processed foods, high sugar intake, and unhealthy fats. The impact of these dietary choices is evident in the rising rates of obesity, type 2 diabetes, and cardiovascular diseases.

Processed foods, often laden with preservatives, additives, and refined sugars, contribute to the caloric excess that underlies obesity—a major risk factor for various chronic conditions. High intake of added sugars, particularly in the form of sugary beverages and snacks, has been linked to insulin resistance, inflammation, and the development of metabolic disorders. Unraveling the complex relationship between dietary choices and chronic diseases involves examining the nutritional quality of foods, understanding the role of macronutrients and micronutrients, and recognizing the importance of dietary patterns in overall health.

The Mediterranean diet, characterized by a high intake of fruits, vegetables, whole grains, and healthy fats, has gained recognition for its potential benefits in preventing chronic diseases. Rich in antioxidants, anti-inflammatory compounds, and essential nutrients, this dietary pattern aligns with principles that promote cardiovascular health, metabolic balance, and overall well-being.

Exploring the impact of dietary choices on chronic illnesses requires a nuanced understanding of individual nutritional needs and cultural influences.

Physical activity, or the lack thereof, stands as another lifestyle factor that profoundly influences health outcomes. The sedentary nature of modern life, marked by increased screen time, desk jobs, and reliance on motorized transportation, contributes to a decline in physical activity levels. Regular physical activity, encompassing activities such as walking, jogging, swimming, and resistance training, not only helps maintain a healthy weight but also plays a direct role in preventing and managing chronic diseases.

The benefits of exercise extend beyond calorie expenditure. Physical activity contributes to improved cardiovascular health by enhancing heart function, regulating blood pressure, and promoting optimal lipid profiles. It also plays a crucial role in glucose metabolism, reducing the risk of type 2 diabetes. Additionally, exercise has profound effects on mental health, with positive impacts on mood, stress management, and cognitive function.

Sedentary behavior, on the other hand, is associated with an increased risk of chronic diseases. Prolonged sitting has been linked to obesity, cardiovascular diseases, and metabolic disorders. Breaking up sedentary time with short bouts of activity, such as standing or stretching, can mitigate these risks. Understanding the relationship between physical activity, sedentary behavior, and chronic illnesses involves exploring the mechanisms through which exercise influences physiological processes and mental well-being.

Sleep, often overlooked in discussions about lifestyle factors, plays a pivotal role in health. The modern pace of life, marked by demanding work schedules, electronic devices, and societal expectations, has led to a prevalence of sleep disturbances. Chronic sleep deprivation or poor sleep quality has been associated with an increased risk of chronic conditions, including obesity, diabetes, cardiovascular diseases, and mental health disorders.

The mechanisms linking sleep and chronic illnesses are multifaceted. Sleep deprivation disrupts hormonal balance, leading to alterations in appetite-regulating hormones and increased cravings for high-calorie foods. It also affects glucose metabolism, insulin sensitivity, and inflammation. Furthermore, inadequate sleep impairs cognitive function, emotional regulation, and overall mental well-being. Recognizing the bidirectional relationship between sleep and chronic diseases is crucial for developing holistic approaches to health promotion.

Stress, a ubiquitous aspect of modern life, represents a significant lifestyle factor that influences health outcomes. Chronic stress, whether related to work, relationships, or other life circumstances, can contribute to the development and exacerbation of chronic illnesses. The physiological response to stress, marked by the release of stress hormones such as cortisol, can lead to systemic inflammation, immune dysfunction, and disruptions in metabolic processes.

The impact of chronic stress on mental health is well-established, with stress being a major contributor to conditions such as anxiety and depression. Additionally, chronic stress has been linked to cardiovascular diseases, gastrointestinal disorders, and autoimmune conditions. Stress

management, therefore, becomes an integral component of lifestyle interventions aimed at preventing and managing chronic diseases.

Mind-body practices, including meditation, mindfulness, and yoga, have gained recognition for their potential in reducing stress and promoting overall well-being. These practices not only help individuals cope with stress but also elicit physiological responses that counteract the negative effects of chronic stress. Exploring the mind-body connection and incorporating stress-reduction techniques into daily life is essential for cultivating resilience and mitigating the impact of stress on health.

Tobacco use, a modifiable lifestyle factor, remains a significant contributor to the burden of chronic diseases. Smoking is a major risk factor for cardiovascular diseases, respiratory conditions such as chronic obstructive pulmonary disease (COPD), and various cancers, including lung cancer. The harmful effects of tobacco extend beyond the smoker to impact those exposed to secondhand smoke.

Addressing tobacco use involves not only individual behavior change but also comprehensive public health strategies. Smoking cessation programs, public awareness campaigns, and policies such as smoke-free environments contribute to reducing the prevalence of tobacco-related chronic diseases. Understanding the social, economic, and cultural factors that influence tobacco use is essential for tailoring interventions to diverse populations.

Alcohol consumption, another lifestyle factor, has complex effects on health depending on the quantity and patterns of use. While moderate alcohol consumption has been associated with certain cardiovascular benefits, excessive alcohol intake poses significant health risks. Chronic alcohol abuse contributes to liver diseases, cardiovascular conditions, neurological disorders, and an increased risk of certain cancers.

The relationship between alcohol and chronic diseases involves intricate interactions with genetic factors, dietary patterns, and overall lifestyle. Recognizing the nuanced impact of alcohol on health, and promoting responsible drinking behaviors, is crucial for preventing the adverse consequences of excessive alcohol consumption. Tailoring public health messages and interventions to consider cultural norms and individual differences is integral to addressing alcohol-related chronic diseases.

Social connections and community engagement represent additional lifestyle factors that influence health outcomes. The quality of social relationships, the strength of social support networks, and the sense of community belonging have all been linked to mental and physical well-being. Conversely, social isolation and loneliness are associated with an increased risk of chronic diseases, including cardiovascular diseases, immune dysfunction, and cognitive decline.

The mechanisms through which social connections influence health are multifaceted. Social support can buffer the effects of stress, provide emotional resilience, and contribute to a sense of purpose and belonging. Community engagement, whether through social, cultural, or recreational activities, fosters a sense of connection and contributes to overall well-being. Recognizing the

importance of social determinants of health is essential for developing interventions that address the broader context in which lifestyle factors operate.

Health disparities, reflecting differences in health outcomes among diverse populations, underscore the need to consider the social determinants of health in discussions about lifestyle factors and chronic diseases. Socioeconomic factors, including income, education, and access to healthcare, influence individuals' ability to make healthy lifestyle choices. Addressing health disparities requires comprehensive strategies that go beyond individual behavior change to consider systemic barriers and inequities.

The life-course perspective, which emphasizes the impact of early-life experiences on health outcomes, is essential for understanding the dynamic nature of lifestyle factors and chronic diseases. Exposures during critical periods of development, such as prenatal and early childhood, can influence the risk of chronic conditions later in life. Recognizing the long-term consequences of early-life experiences informs interventions that promote health across the lifespan.

Lifestyle factors are integral determinants of health, playing a central role in the development, prevention, and management of chronic diseases. From dietary choices and physical activity levels to sleep patterns, stress management, and social connections, lifestyle factors influence the intricate web of factors that contribute to health outcomes. Recognizing the multidimensional nature of lifestyle and its interactions with genetic predispositions, environmental triggers, and social determinants is essential for developing holistic approaches to health promotion. Empowering individuals to make informed choices about their lifestyles, addressing systemic barriers to health, and fostering supportive environments contribute to a comprehensive strategy for navigating the pathways to health and preventing the burden of chronic diseases.

CHAPTER TWO

Inflammation's Role in Chronic Disease

In the intricate landscape of chronic diseases, inflammation emerges as a central player, weaving its intricate threads through a multitude of health conditions. Once regarded simply as a response to injury or infection, inflammation is now recognized as a dynamic and complex process that, when chronic and dysregulated, can contribute to the development and progression of a wide array of chronic illnesses. Understanding the nuances of inflammation's role in chronic disease requires delving into the molecular and cellular mechanisms, exploring the diverse conditions influenced by inflammation, and unraveling the intricate web of factors that contribute to chronic inflammatory states.

At its core, inflammation is a natural and essential part of the body's defense mechanism. When the body detects injury or infection, a cascade of events is set in motion to protect tissues, eliminate pathogens, and facilitate the healing process. Acute inflammation is a tightly regulated and self-limiting response that serves a protective role. However, when inflammation becomes chronic, persisting over an extended period, it can shift from a beneficial process to a driving force behind many chronic diseases.

The molecular and cellular players in inflammation orchestrate a complex symphony. The process involves immune cells, signaling molecules, and a series of tightly regulated events. One key player is the immune system's white blood cells, which include neutrophils, macrophages, and lymphocytes. These cells migrate to the site of injury or infection, releasing a variety of signaling molecules known as cytokines. These cytokines communicate with other cells, amplifying the immune response and contributing to the inflammatory cascade.

In chronic inflammation, this finely tuned orchestra of immune responses becomes dysregulated. The immune system may be activated persistently, even in the absence of a clear threat. This sustained activation can lead to a continuous release of pro-inflammatory cytokines, such as tumor necrosis factor-alpha (TNF-alpha), interleukin-6 (IL-6), and interleukin-1 beta (IL-1β). These molecules, in turn, can perpetuate inflammation, creating a self-sustaining loop that contributes to tissue damage and the pathogenesis of chronic diseases.

Atherosclerosis, the buildup of plaques in the arteries, exemplifies the intricate relationship between inflammation and chronic diseases. Initially considered a disorder primarily driven by elevated cholesterol levels, atherosclerosis is now recognized as an inflammatory condition. The inflammatory process plays a crucial role in the initiation and progression of atherosclerotic plaques. Endothelial cells lining the arteries undergo dysfunction, allowing immune cells to infiltrate the vessel walls. These immune cells, particularly macrophages, engulf cholesterol particles, forming foam cells that contribute to plaque formation. The inflammation within these plaques further promotes a cascade of events leading to plaque instability and rupture, ultimately culminating in cardiovascular events such as heart attacks and strokes.

Chronic inflammatory states are intimately linked to metabolic disorders, with obesity standing at the crossroads of inflammation and metabolic dysregulation. Adipose tissue, once viewed solely as a passive energy storage depot, is now recognized as an active endocrine organ capable of secreting pro-inflammatory molecules. In obesity, the expansion of adipose tissue triggers an immune response, recruiting macrophages and other immune cells. This immune cell infiltration results in the release of inflammatory cytokines and contributes to insulin resistance, a key feature of type 2 diabetes.

The relationship between inflammation and diabetes extends beyond insulin resistance. Chronic inflammation has been implicated in the dysfunction of pancreatic beta cells, which produce insulin. Additionally, inflammation plays a role in the complications of diabetes, contributing to cardiovascular diseases, kidney damage, and peripheral neuropathy. The intricate interplay between inflammation and metabolic disorders underscores the systemic nature of chronic inflammatory states and their impact on various aspects of health.

Autoimmune diseases, a diverse group of conditions where the immune system mistakenly attacks the body's own tissues, exemplify the dysregulation of immune responses that underlies chronic inflammation. Rheumatoid arthritis, an autoimmune disorder affecting the joints, showcases the role of inflammation in tissue destruction. In rheumatoid arthritis, the immune system targets the synovium, the lining of the joints, leading to chronic inflammation, pain, and joint damage.

Systemic lupus erythematosus (SLE), another autoimmune condition, demonstrates the systemic effects of chronic inflammation. In SLE, the immune system can attack multiple organs and tissues, including the skin, joints, kidneys, and cardiovascular system. The inflammatory response in SLE contributes to a range of symptoms, from rashes and joint pain to kidney dysfunction and an increased risk of cardiovascular events.

Inflammatory bowel diseases (IBD), including Crohn's disease and ulcerative colitis, exemplify the impact of chronic inflammation on the gastrointestinal system. In these conditions, the immune system mistakenly targets the digestive tract, leading to persistent inflammation and damage to the intestinal lining. The consequences include symptoms such as abdominal pain, diarrhea, and weight loss, as well as complications such as strictures and fistulas.

Neurodegenerative disorders, such as Alzheimer's and Parkinson's diseases, also have inflammatory components contributing to their pathogenesis. In Alzheimer's disease, chronic inflammation in the brain is characterized by the presence of immune cells and inflammatory molecules. This neuroinflammation is believed to contribute to the accumulation of abnormal protein aggregates, such as beta-amyloid plaques and tau tangles, which are hallmarks of the disease.

In Parkinson's disease, inflammation is implicated in the progressive loss of dopaminergic neurons. The activation of microglia, the immune cells of the central nervous system, contributes to the release of inflammatory mediators, contributing to neuronal damage. The intricate interplay between inflammation and neurodegenerative processes highlights the complexity of chronic diseases that affect the nervous system.

Cancer, a multifaceted group of diseases characterized by uncontrolled cell growth, is intricately linked to inflammation. Chronic inflammation contributes to the initiation, promotion, and progression of various cancers. The inflammatory microenvironment within tumors can facilitate angiogenesis, promote tumor cell survival, and contribute to metastasis—the spread of cancer to other parts of the body.

The link between inflammation and cancer is evident in conditions such as inflammatory bowel disease-associated colorectal cancer and hepatitis C virus-induced liver cancer. Inflammatory processes contribute to DNA damage, genetic mutations, and alterations in the tissue microenvironment, creating an environment conducive to the development of malignancies. Recognizing the role of chronic inflammation in cancer underscores the potential for anti-inflammatory strategies in cancer prevention and treatment.

The gut, often referred to as the "second brain" due to its complex neural network, represents a unique interface between the external environment and the immune system. The gut microbiota, a diverse community of microorganisms inhabiting the gastrointestinal tract, plays a pivotal role in maintaining gut health and modulating immune responses. Disruptions in the balance of the gut microbiota, known as dysbiosis, can contribute to chronic inflammation and the development of various diseases.

Inflammatory bowel diseases, irritable bowel syndrome, and celiac disease are examples of conditions where the interplay between the gut, the microbiota, and the immune system is central to pathogenesis. In these disorders, factors such as genetic predisposition, environmental triggers, and alterations in the gut microbiota contribute to chronic inflammatory states. Understanding the intricate relationship between the gut and inflammation opens avenues for therapeutic interventions targeting the microbiome to modulate immune responses and promote health.

The role of lifestyle factors in influencing inflammation adds another layer of complexity to the understanding of chronic diseases. Diet, for instance, plays a crucial role in shaping the inflammatory milieu within the body. The Western diet, characterized by high levels of processed foods, saturated fats, and sugars, is associated with elevated inflammatory markers. In contrast, anti-inflammatory diets, such as the Mediterranean diet, emphasize whole foods, fruits, vegetables, and healthy fats, and have been linked to reduced inflammation and a lower risk of chronic diseases.

Physical activity, a well-established modulator of immune function, also influences inflammation. Regular exercise has anti-inflammatory effects, reducing levels of pro-inflammatory cytokines and promoting a balanced immune response. Conversely, sedentary behavior and obesity are associated with chronic low-grade inflammation, contributing to the development of metabolic disorders and cardiovascular diseases.

Sleep, a fundamental aspect of lifestyle, has bidirectional interactions with inflammation. Chronic sleep deprivation and poor sleep quality can promote inflammation, while inflammation, in turn, can disrupt sleep patterns. The complex interplay between sleep and inflammation highlights the importance of addressing sleep hygiene as part of comprehensive strategies for managing chronic diseases.

Stress, another lifestyle factor, is intricately linked to inflammation. Chronic stress activates the immune system, leading to the release of pro-inflammatory molecules. Stress-induced inflammation has been implicated in various chronic conditions, including cardiovascular diseases, mental health disorders, and autoimmune diseases. Mind-body practices, such as meditation and mindfulness, offer potential avenues for mitigating stress-related inflammation and promoting overall well-being.

Environmental factors, ranging from pollutants and toxins to infectious agents, also contribute to chronic inflammation. Air pollution, for example, exposes individuals to particulate matter and airborne toxins that can trigger inflammatory responses in the respiratory system and have systemic effects. Chronic exposure to environmental pollutants has been linked to respiratory conditions, cardiovascular diseases, and other inflammatory disorders.

Genetics, too, plays a role in shaping individual susceptibility to inflammation and chronic diseases. Genetic variations can influence the regulation of immune responses and the balance between pro-inflammatory and anti-inflammatory pathways. Understanding the interplay between genetics and inflammation provides insights into personalized approaches for disease prevention and treatment.

Therapeutic strategies targeting inflammation have shown promise in managing chronic diseases. Nonsteroidal anti-inflammatory drugs (NSAIDs), corticosteroids, and disease-modifying antirheumatic drugs (DMARDs) are examples of medications used to control inflammation in conditions such as rheumatoid arthritis and inflammatory bowel diseases. Biologic agents, which specifically target inflammatory molecules, have revolutionized the treatment landscape for various autoimmune diseases.

Lifestyle interventions also offer avenues for modulating inflammation and promoting health. Dietary modifications, such as adopting an anti-inflammatory diet rich in fruits, vegetables, and omega-3 fatty acids, have been associated with reduced inflammatory markers. Regular physical activity, weight management, and stress reduction strategies contribute to an anti-inflammatory lifestyle. Integrative approaches, including complementary and alternative therapies, explore the potential of natural compounds and mind-body practices in modulating inflammation.

The gut microbiome, with its intricate relationship to inflammation, represents a novel target for therapeutic interventions. Probiotics, prebiotics, and fecal microbiota transplantation are emerging as strategies to modulate the gut microbiota and influence immune responses. The potential for microbiome-targeted therapies to impact various chronic diseases underscores the importance of understanding the gut-immune axis in health and disease.

Precision medicine, an evolving paradigm in healthcare, seeks to tailor interventions based on individual genetic, environmental, and lifestyle factors. In the context of inflammation and chronic diseases, precision medicine holds the promise of personalized treatment plans that target the specific pathways driving inflammation in each individual. Biomarkers indicative of inflammatory states and genetic profiles may guide the selection of therapies tailored to an individual's unique needs.

The intricate web of inflammation's role in chronic disease emphasizes the need for a holistic and interdisciplinary approach to healthcare. Recognizing inflammation as a common denominator across diverse conditions opens new avenues for shared therapeutic strategies. Integrating lifestyle modifications, environmental interventions, and targeted therapies offers a comprehensive framework for managing chronic diseases at their inflammatory roots.

Preventive strategies, rooted in the understanding of inflammation, extend beyond the realm of treatment. Public health initiatives that address the determinants of chronic inflammation, including lifestyle factors, environmental exposures, and social determinants of health, contribute to a broader strategy for disease prevention. Education, awareness, and policy changes that promote anti-inflammatory lifestyles and create supportive environments are essential components of population-wide efforts to reduce the burden of chronic diseases.

Inflammation's role in chronic disease represents a dynamic and multifaceted aspect of health. From the molecular and cellular mechanisms to the diverse array of conditions influenced by inflammation, the complex interplay between the immune system and chronic diseases requires a nuanced understanding. Exploring the intricate web of factors contributing to chronic inflammatory states opens avenues for therapeutic interventions and preventive strategies that address the root causes of diverse health conditions. As we unravel the complexities of inflammation in chronic diseases, a holistic approach that integrates medical, lifestyle, and environmental perspectives paves the way for a future where the inflammatory landscape is understood, modulated, and ultimately harnessed for the promotion of health and well-being.

Identifying and Addressing Chronic Inflammatory Processes

Chronic inflammatory processes weave their influence, contributing to the development and progression of a myriad of conditions. Recognizing and understanding these persistent inflammatory states is essential for developing effective strategies to prevent, manage, and treat chronic diseases. This exploration delves into the mechanisms of chronic inflammation, highlights the diverse conditions associated with it, and outlines a comprehensive approach to identify and address these inflammatory processes for the betterment of individual and public health.

The Underlying Mechanisms of Chronic Inflammation

Inflammation is a fundamental aspect of the body's defense system, designed to protect against injuries, infections, and other threats to tissue integrity. In its acute form, inflammation is a temporary and localized response that promotes healing and recovery. However, when inflammation becomes chronic, lasting for an extended period and often manifesting systemically, it can contribute to a range of health issues.

The molecular and cellular processes involved in chronic inflammation are intricate and multifaceted. Immune cells, particularly macrophages, play a central role in perpetuating inflammatory responses. These cells release a cascade of signaling molecules known as cytokines, including tumor necrosis factor-alpha (TNF-alpha), interleukin-6 (IL-6), and interleukin-1 beta (IL-1β). Chronic activation of immune cells and sustained release of pro-inflammatory cytokines create a state of persistent inflammation.

Underlying chronic inflammatory processes are often dysregulations in the intricate balance between pro-inflammatory and anti-inflammatory signals. The body's inability to resolve inflammation appropriately can result from various factors, including genetic predispositions, environmental exposures, and lifestyle choices. Genetic variations in immune system genes, for instance, can influence an individual's susceptibility to chronic inflammation, highlighting the role of personalized medicine in understanding and addressing these processes.

The Diverse Landscape of Conditions Associated with Chronic Inflammation

Chronic inflammatory processes are not confined to a specific set of diseases; rather, they permeate a wide range of health conditions. Understanding the diverse landscape of conditions associated with chronic inflammation is crucial for developing targeted interventions. Some of the prominent areas where chronic inflammation plays a pivotal role include:

Cardiovascular Diseases

Atherosclerosis, the process of plaque buildup in arteries, is intricately linked to chronic inflammation. In response to endothelial dysfunction, immune cells infiltrate arterial walls, setting off an inflammatory cascade that contributes to the formation and progression of atherosclerotic plaques. These plaques can rupture, triggering blood clot formation and leading to heart attacks and strokes.

Metabolic Disorders

Chronic inflammation is closely intertwined with metabolic dysregulation, particularly in the context of obesity and type 2 diabetes. Adipose tissue, once considered a passive storage depot, becomes an active contributor to inflammation in obesity. The resulting insulin resistance, driven by chronic low-grade inflammation, is a hallmark of type 2 diabetes.

Autoimmune Diseases

Conditions such as rheumatoid arthritis, lupus, and inflammatory bowel diseases are characterized by dysregulated immune responses that lead to chronic inflammation. In autoimmune disorders, the immune system mistakenly targets the body's own tissues, setting off a cascade of inflammatory processes that contribute to tissue damage.

Neurodegenerative Disorders

Chronic inflammation is implicated in the pathogenesis of neurodegenerative diseases like Alzheimer's and Parkinson's. In Alzheimer's disease, neuroinflammation accompanies the accumulation of abnormal protein aggregates in the brain. Similarly, in Parkinson's disease, chronic inflammation contributes to the loss of dopaminergic neurons.

Cancer

The relationship between inflammation and cancer is intricate and bidirectional. Chronic inflammation creates a microenvironment conducive to cancer development, promoting cell proliferation, angiogenesis, and metastasis. Conversely, cancer cells can release signals that attract immune cells, perpetuating an inflammatory milieu.

Gastrointestinal Conditions

Inflammatory bowel diseases, including Crohn's disease and ulcerative colitis, are characterized by chronic inflammation of the gastrointestinal tract. The immune system's misdirected attacks on the gut lining result in persistent inflammation, causing symptoms such as abdominal pain, diarrhea, and weight loss.

Identifying Chronic Inflammatory Processes

The challenge in addressing chronic inflammatory processes lies in their often subtle and insidious nature. Unlike acute inflammation, which manifests with overt signs like redness, swelling, and pain, chronic inflammation can be asymptomatic or present with nonspecific symptoms. Robust diagnostic strategies are, therefore, crucial for identifying and characterizing chronic inflammatory processes.

Biomarkers of Inflammation

Several biomarkers serve as indicators of systemic inflammation. C-reactive protein (CRP), an acute-phase protein produced by the liver, is a widely used marker of inflammation. Elevated levels of CRP are associated with an increased risk of cardiovascular events and are indicative of systemic inflammation. Other biomarkers, such as erythrocyte sedimentation rate (ESR) and certain cytokines, can also provide insights into the inflammatory status.

Imaging Techniques

Advanced imaging technologies, including positron emission tomography (PET) scans and magnetic resonance imaging (MRI), enable visualization of inflammatory processes within tissues. These imaging modalities can be particularly valuable in assessing conditions where chronic inflammation is a contributing factor, such as rheumatoid arthritis or atherosclerosis.

Genetic Profiling

Understanding an individual's genetic predisposition to inflammation can be instrumental in identifying those at higher risk for chronic inflammatory conditions. Genetic profiling allows for the identification of variations in genes associated with immune function and inflammation, contributing to personalized approaches in healthcare.

Comprehensive Health Assessments

Assessing overall health through comprehensive evaluations, including metabolic panels, lipid profiles, and assessments of organ function, provides a holistic view of an individual's well-being. Chronic inflammatory processes often leave metabolic imprints that can be detected through such assessments.

Patient-reported Symptoms

Considering the subjective experiences reported by individuals is essential in the diagnostic process. Symptoms such as fatigue, joint pain, and recurrent infections may be indicative of underlying chronic inflammatory conditions. Collecting a thorough medical history and paying attention to patient-reported symptoms contribute to a more nuanced understanding of inflammatory states.

Addressing Chronic Inflammatory Processes: A Multifaceted Approach

Once identified, addressing chronic inflammatory processes necessitates a comprehensive and multifaceted approach. This approach should encompass lifestyle modifications, targeted therapies, and interventions aimed at modulating the underlying causes of inflammation. Key components of this approach include:

Lifestyle Modifications

- Dietary Interventions: Adopting an anti-inflammatory diet can play a pivotal role in managing chronic inflammatory processes. Emphasizing whole foods, such as fruits, vegetables, nuts, and fatty fish, while reducing processed foods, sugars, and unhealthy fats, helps create a dietary environment that supports overall health.
- Physical Activity: Regular exercise is a potent modulator of inflammation. Physical activity has been shown to reduce levels of pro-inflammatory cytokines while promoting the release of anti-inflammatory molecules. Incorporating both aerobic and resistance exercises into a routine contributes to the overall anti-inflammatory effect.

- Stress Management: Chronic stress is a significant contributor to inflammation. Implementing stress management techniques, such as mindfulness, meditation, and relaxation exercises, can help regulate the body's stress response and mitigate chronic inflammatory states.
- Adequate Sleep: Prioritizing sufficient and quality sleep is crucial for maintaining health and regulating inflammation. Chronic sleep deprivation and poor sleep quality can contribute to systemic inflammation, emphasizing the importance of cultivating healthy sleep habits.

Pharmacological Interventions

- Nonsteroidal Anti-inflammatory Drugs (NSAIDs): NSAIDs, including aspirin and ibuprofen, are commonly used to alleviate symptoms of inflammation. While effective for managing acute inflammatory conditions, their long-term use may be limited by potential side effects.
- Biologic Therapies: Biologic drugs, designed to target specific molecules involved in the inflammatory cascade, have revolutionized the treatment of conditions such as rheumatoid arthritis, psoriasis, and inflammatory bowel diseases. These targeted therapies aim to interrupt the inflammatory processes at the molecular level.
- Immunomodulatory Agents: Drugs that modulate the immune system, such as corticosteroids and disease-modifying antirheumatic drugs (DMARDs), are employed in conditions where chronic inflammation is driven by autoimmune responses. These medications help regulate immune activity and reduce inflammation.

Integrative and Complementary Therapies

- Nutraceuticals: Certain dietary supplements, known as nutraceuticals, have demonstrated anti-inflammatory properties. Omega-3 fatty acids, found in fish oil, and curcumin, derived from turmeric, are examples of nutraceuticals with potential anti-inflammatory effects.
- Herbal Remedies: Herbal remedies from traditional medicine systems, such as Ayurveda and Traditional Chinese Medicine, may offer natural anti-inflammatory benefits. Compounds derived from herbs like ginger, boswellia, and green tea have shown promise in modulating inflammatory responses.

- Mind-Body Practices: Practices that integrate the mind and body, such as yoga and tai chi, have been associated with anti-inflammatory effects. These activities not only promote physical well-being but also contribute to stress reduction and overall mental health.

Gut Health Interventions

- Probiotics: Probiotics, live microorganisms that confer health benefits, play a role in modulating gut microbiota and influencing immune responses. Incorporating probiotic-rich foods or supplements may contribute to a balanced gut microbiome and help manage inflammation.
- Prebiotics: Prebiotics are substances that promote the growth of beneficial microorganisms in the gut. Dietary fibers, found in fruits, vegetables, and whole grains, serve as prebiotics, fostering an environment conducive to gut health.
- Microbiota Transplantation: Fecal microbiota transplantation (FMT) involves transferring healthy gut bacteria from a donor to a recipient. While primarily utilized in conditions like Clostridioides difficile infection, emerging research explores its potential in modulating inflammatory responses in other contexts.

Precision Medicine Approaches

- Genomic Medicine: Understanding the genetic basis of inflammatory processes allows for personalized interventions. Genomic medicine, which involves tailoring treatments based on an individual's genetic makeup, holds promise in identifying optimal therapeutic approaches for managing chronic inflammatory conditions.
- Biomarker-guided Therapy: Biomarkers indicative of inflammatory states can guide the selection and monitoring of therapeutic interventions. Tailoring treatments based on the specific inflammatory profile of an individual enhances the precision and effectiveness of interventions.

The Role of Public Health and Policy

Addressing chronic inflammatory processes extends beyond individual healthcare to encompass broader public health and policy initiatives. Creating environments that support anti-inflammatory lifestyles and addressing social determinants of health contribute to population-wide efforts. Key elements of this approach include:

Health Education and Awareness

Public health campaigns that educate individuals about the impact of lifestyle choices on inflammation and overall health are crucial. Raising awareness about the role of chronic

inflammation in various diseases empowers individuals to make informed decisions about their lifestyles.

Access to Healthy Food and Physical Activity

Policy measures that improve access to healthy food options and promote physical activity contribute to population-wide inflammation management. Initiatives such as community gardens, urban planning for walkability, and subsidizing healthy foods in underserved areas address the social determinants of health.

Environmental Protection

Mitigating environmental factors that contribute to chronic inflammation requires robust environmental protection policies. Regulations aimed at reducing air and water pollution, controlling exposure to toxins, and promoting sustainable practices contribute to a healthier environment and reduced inflammatory burdens.

Reducing Health Disparities

Addressing health disparities involves recognizing and addressing the systemic factors that contribute to differential health outcomes among diverse populations. Policies that ensure equitable access to healthcare, education, and economic opportunities contribute to reducing disparities in inflammatory health.

Research and Innovation

Investing in research that deepens our understanding of chronic inflammatory processes and identifies novel interventions is vital. Research initiatives exploring the intersection of genomics, microbiomics, and immunology contribute to the development of innovative therapies and preventive strategies.

Challenges and Future Directions

While progress has been made in understanding and addressing chronic inflammatory processes, challenges remain. Identifying reliable biomarkers that accurately reflect the complex and dynamic nature of inflammation poses a persistent challenge. The heterogeneity of inflammatory responses among individuals further complicates the development of universal diagnostic and therapeutic approaches.

The integration of various interventions, including lifestyle modifications, pharmacological therapies, and complementary approaches, necessitates a holistic and patient-centered approach to care. Implementing such multifaceted interventions within existing healthcare systems requires collaboration among healthcare providers, researchers, policymakers, and the community.

The role of individual variability, including genetic factors and the unique microbiome composition of each individual, underscores the need for precision medicine approaches. Tailoring interventions based on an individual's specific inflammatory profile holds promise in optimizing treatment outcomes and minimizing potential side effects.

Looking ahead, technological advancements, including the application of artificial intelligence and big data analytics, offer opportunities to enhance our understanding of chronic inflammatory processes. Integrating these technologies into healthcare systems can enable more personalized and data-driven approaches to inflammation management.

Identifying and addressing chronic inflammatory processes represents a dynamic and evolving frontier in healthcare. From the molecular intricacies of immune responses to the diverse array of conditions influenced by chronic inflammation, a comprehensive approach is essential. By recognizing the multifaceted nature of chronic inflammatory states and implementing strategies that span lifestyle modifications, targeted therapies, and public health initiatives, we pave the way for a future where the impact of inflammation on health is understood, managed, and ultimately minimized. As we navigate this complex landscape, a commitment to interdisciplinary collaboration, research innovation, and personalized approaches ensures a holistic and effective strategy for promoting inflammatory health and overall well-being.

CHAPTER THREE

Gut Microbiota and Health: Nurturing the Microbial Allies Within

The human gut is a bustling ecosystem teeming with trillions of microorganisms, collectively known as the gut microbiota. This intricate community of bacteria, viruses, fungi, and other microorganisms plays a pivotal role in maintaining health and influencing various physiological processes. The dynamic interplay between the host and the gut microbiota extends far beyond digestion, impacting immune function, metabolism, and even mental health. As we delve into the complexities of the gut microbiota, a fascinating journey unfolds, revealing the symbiotic relationship between these microbial allies and our overall well-being.

The Microbial Symphony: Understanding the Gut Microbiota

The gut microbiota is a diverse and dynamic community residing in the gastrointestinal tract, with the majority of its members residing in the colon. Comprising trillions of microorganisms, the gut microbiota collectively harbors a vast array of species, each contributing to the overall microbial balance. The composition of the gut microbiota is influenced by various factors, including genetics, diet, lifestyle, and environmental exposures.

Bacteria are the predominant members of the gut microbiota, with thousands of different species identified. Among them, the two major phyla, Firmicutes and Bacteroidetes, dominate the landscape. Actinobacteria, Proteobacteria, and Verrucomicrobia are also present, albeit in smaller proportions. This intricate balance of microbial species forms a complex ecosystem, akin to a microbial orchestra where each member plays a unique role.

Beyond bacteria, the gut microbiota includes viruses (bacteriophages), fungi (eukaryotes), and archaea. Bacteriophages, viruses that infect bacteria, contribute to the regulation of bacterial populations. Fungi, such as Candida and Saccharomyces, coexist with bacteria, while archaea, although less abundant, play a role in microbial metabolism.

Early Life Seeding: The Influence of Birth and Breastfeeding

The initial colonization of the gut begins at birth, with the mode of delivery influencing the types of microbes a newborn encounters. Infants born vaginally acquire a microbiota resembling that of the mother's vaginal and fecal microbiota, while those born via Cesarean section show a microbiota more reflective of the skin and environmental microbes.

Breastfeeding further shapes the infant's gut microbiota. Breast milk contains an array of bioactive compounds, including prebiotics that serve as nourishment for beneficial bacteria. Bifidobacteria, in particular, thrive on the oligosaccharides present in breast milk, contributing to the establishment of a healthy gut microbiota.

The early years of life represent a critical window for gut microbiota development. This period of microbial seeding and maturation establishes the foundation for the individual's gut microbiota composition, influencing health outcomes throughout life.

Gut Microbiota and Immune Harmony

The gut microbiota and the immune system engage in a complex dance, maintaining a delicate balance between defense against pathogens and tolerance to beneficial microbes. The gut-associated lymphoid tissue (GALT), a significant component of the immune system located in the gastrointestinal tract, plays a pivotal role in orchestrating immune responses in the presence of the gut microbiota.

Beneficial bacteria within the gut microbiota contribute to immune tolerance by promoting the development of regulatory T cells. These specialized immune cells play a crucial role in preventing inappropriate immune responses, reducing the risk of autoimmune conditions where the immune system mistakenly targets the body's own tissues.

Conversely, the gut microbiota serves as a formidable barrier against pathogenic invaders. Beneficial bacteria compete for resources and produce antimicrobial peptides, creating an environment unfavorable for harmful microorganisms. This competitive exclusion helps protect against infections and reinforces the first line of defense provided by the mucosal surfaces of the gastrointestinal tract.

Metabolic Harmony: Gut Microbiota and Host Metabolism

The gut microbiota is intricately linked to host metabolism, influencing energy extraction, nutrient absorption, and even the storage of fat. The fermentation of dietary fibers by certain gut bacteria produces short-chain fatty acids (SCFAs), which serve as an energy source for the cells lining the colon and play a role in metabolic regulation.

Bile acids, essential for fat digestion and absorption, undergo modifications by gut bacteria, influencing their signaling properties. This interaction between the gut microbiota and bile acids affects metabolic processes, including lipid metabolism and glucose homeostasis.

Imbalances in the gut microbiota, such as a reduction in microbial diversity or an overgrowth of harmful bacteria, have been associated with metabolic disorders. Conditions like obesity and type 2 diabetes show alterations in the gut microbiota composition, highlighting the potential role of microbial dysbiosis in metabolic disturbances.

The Brain-Gut Axis: Influence on Mental Health

The intricate communication network between the gut and the brain, known as the brain-gut axis, underscores the bidirectional relationship between the gut microbiota and mental health. Emerging research has revealed that the gut microbiota can influence brain function and behavior, with implications for conditions such as anxiety, depression, and stress.

The gut microbiota produces neurotransmitters, such as serotonin and gamma-aminobutyric acid (GABA), which are involved in mood regulation. Serotonin, in particular, plays a crucial role in emotional well-being, and alterations in its levels have been linked to mood disorders.

Microbial metabolites, including SCFAs, also play a role in brain health. SCFAs can cross the blood-brain barrier and influence the activity of microglia, the immune cells of the central nervous system. This interaction between microbial metabolites and the brain's immune cells contributes to neuroinflammation and may impact cognitive function.

Dysregulation of the brain-gut axis has been implicated in conditions such as irritable bowel syndrome (IBS), where gastrointestinal symptoms are often accompanied by alterations in mood and stress responses. The intricate interplay between the gut microbiota and the brain highlights the holistic nature of health, where the gut's microbial residents contribute to mental well-being.

Dysbiosis: Disruptions in Gut Microbiota Harmony

Dysbiosis, an imbalance or disruption in the gut microbiota composition, is associated with various health conditions. It can result from factors such as antibiotic use, dietary changes, stress, and infections. Dysbiosis is characterized by a reduction in microbial diversity, alterations in the relative abundance of specific bacteria, and the potential overgrowth of harmful microorganisms.

Inflammatory bowel diseases (IBD), including Crohn's disease and ulcerative colitis, are examples where dysbiosis is implicated in disease pathogenesis. The altered gut microbiota in individuals with IBD may contribute to chronic inflammation and the characteristic symptoms of these conditions, including abdominal pain, diarrhea, and weight loss.

Conditions like irritable bowel syndrome (IBS), characterized by gastrointestinal symptoms without identifiable structural abnormalities, also show associations with dysbiosis. Changes in

the abundance of certain bacterial species, along with alterations in microbial metabolites, may contribute to the symptoms experienced by individuals with IBS.

Nurturing a Healthy Gut Microbiota: Dietary and Lifestyle Influences

The composition of the gut microbiota is highly responsive to dietary and lifestyle factors, offering avenues for individuals to positively influence their microbial allies. A diet rich in fiber, found in fruits, vegetables, whole grains, and legumes, promotes the growth of beneficial bacteria that thrive on these dietary fibers.

Prebiotics, non-digestible fibers that serve as food for beneficial bacteria, can be incorporated into the diet to support the growth of specific microbial species. Examples of prebiotic-rich foods include garlic, onions, leeks, asparagus, and bananas.

Probiotics, live microorganisms with health benefits when consumed in adequate amounts, are another tool for promoting gut health. Fermented foods, such as yogurt, kefir, sauerkraut, and kimchi, contain beneficial bacteria that can contribute to the diversity and balance of the gut microbiota.

Polyphenol-rich foods, including berries, tea, and dark chocolate, have been associated with positive effects on the gut microbiota. These bioactive compounds, found in plant-based foods, may have prebiotic-like effects, supporting the growth of beneficial bacteria.

Regular physical activity has been linked to a more diverse and resilient gut microbiota. Exercise appears to promote microbial diversity and the abundance of beneficial bacteria, contributing to overall gut health.

Adequate sleep is essential for maintaining a healthy gut microbiota. Disruptions in sleep patterns or chronic sleep deprivation have been associated with alterations in the gut microbiota composition, highlighting the importance of prioritizing quality sleep for overall well-being.

Reducing stress through mindfulness practices, meditation, and relaxation techniques can positively influence the gut microbiota. Chronic stress is known to impact the gut-brain axis and may contribute to dysbiosis, emphasizing the need for stress management strategies.

Antibiotics and the Gut Microbiota: Navigating the Impact

Antibiotics, while invaluable in treating bacterial infections, can have a significant impact on the gut microbiota. These medications do not discriminate between harmful and beneficial bacteria, leading to alterations in microbial composition and diversity.

The use of broad-spectrum antibiotics, which target a wide range of bacteria, can result in more profound changes in the gut microbiota. This disruption may pave the way for opportunistic

pathogens to flourish and contribute to conditions such as Clostridium difficile infection, a bacterial overgrowth associated with antibiotic use.

Probiotics, taken concurrently with antibiotics or during the recovery period, can help restore microbial balance. These beneficial microorganisms can aid in preventing the overgrowth of harmful bacteria and support the reestablishment of a diverse and resilient gut microbiota.

Therapeutic Potential: Manipulating the Gut Microbiota

The therapeutic potential of modulating the gut microbiota is a burgeoning area of research, offering innovative approaches to various health conditions. Fecal microbiota transplantation (FMT), a procedure where fecal material from a healthy donor is transferred to the gut of an individual with dysbiosis, has shown remarkable success in treating recurrent Clostridium difficile infection.

Microbial-based therapies, including the use of specific bacteria or microbial consortia, are being explored for conditions such as inflammatory bowel diseases and irritable bowel syndrome. The goal is to restore microbial balance and promote a healthy gut environment.

Precision medicine approaches aim to tailor interventions based on an individual's unique gut microbiota profile. By understanding an individual's microbial composition, personalized dietary recommendations, probiotic formulations, or microbial-based therapies can be designed to target specific imbalances.

The Gut Microbiota in Disease: From Associations to Causation

Associations between alterations in the gut microbiota and various diseases have been extensively documented. However, establishing causation—determining whether changes in the gut microbiota contribute to disease development or are a consequence of the disease—remains a complex challenge.

Research is ongoing to unravel the intricate relationships between the gut microbiota and conditions such as obesity, diabetes, autoimmune diseases, and mental health disorders. Understanding the mechanisms by which the gut microbiota influences these conditions opens avenues for targeted interventions and therapeutic strategies.

Challenges and Future Directions

Despite the growing understanding of the gut microbiota's impact on health, challenges persist in unraveling its complexities. Interindividual variability, influenced by genetics, lifestyle, and environmental factors, adds layers of complexity to studying the gut microbiota's role in health and disease.

Standardizing methodologies for studying the gut microbiota, including sample collection, DNA sequencing, and data analysis, is essential for comparing research findings across studies. Advances in technology, such as high-throughput sequencing and metagenomic analysis, continue to enhance our ability to characterize the gut microbiota with greater precision.

The role of the gut microbiota in personalized medicine is a promising frontier. Tailoring interventions based on an individual's unique microbial profile has the potential to optimize treatment outcomes and enhance therapeutic efficacy.

Public health initiatives that promote gut health awareness and provide education on the importance of a balanced and diverse diet are essential. Integrating gut health considerations into dietary guidelines and healthcare practices contributes to a holistic approach to well-being.

Cultivating a Symbiotic Relationship

The journey through the intricate landscape of the gut microbiota reveals a symbiotic relationship that extends far beyond digestion. From the moment of birth, the gut microbiota becomes a lifelong companion, influencing health outcomes across the lifespan. As we unlock the secrets of this microbial world, the potential for innovative therapies, preventive strategies, and personalized approaches to health beckons.

Cultivating a symbiotic relationship with the gut microbiota involves nurturing microbial allies through mindful dietary choices, lifestyle practices, and a deeper understanding of the factors that shape microbial harmony. The gut microbiota, with its vast diversity and functional richness, is a testament to the interconnectedness of human health and the microbial world within.

In embracing the wisdom of this microbial symphony, we embark on a journey of discovery, where the profound impact of the gut microbiota on health opens new horizons for medical science and individual well-being.

Microbial Dysbiosis in Chronic Conditions

Microbial dysbiosis, an imbalance in the composition and function of the microbiota, has emerged as a critical factor in the development and progression of various chronic conditions. The human body hosts a vast array of microorganisms, collectively known as the microbiota, which play a crucial role in maintaining homeostasis and supporting essential physiological functions. When this delicate balance is disrupted, microbial dysbiosis can ensue, contributing to the pathogenesis of chronic diseases. This comprehensive exploration delves into the mechanisms, implications, and potential therapeutic interventions associated with microbial dysbiosis in chronic conditions.

The Human Microbiota: A Dynamic Ecosystem

The human microbiota is a dynamic ecosystem comprising trillions of microorganisms, including bacteria, viruses, fungi, and archaea, inhabiting various niches such as the skin, gastrointestinal tract, oral cavity, and respiratory system. The gut microbiota, in particular, has garnered significant attention due to its pivotal role in digestion, nutrient absorption, immune modulation, and protection against pathogenic invaders. The delicate balance within this microbial community is essential for maintaining health, and disruptions can lead to microbial dysbiosis.

Microbial Dysbiosis: Underlying Mechanisms

Understanding the mechanisms underlying microbial dysbiosis is crucial for unraveling its role in chronic conditions. Several factors contribute to the disruption of the microbiota equilibrium, including:

1. Dietary Factors:

   - The composition of the microbiota is highly influenced by dietary patterns.

   - High-fat, low-fiber diets are associated with alterations in microbial diversity, favoring the growth of pro-inflammatory species.

2. Antibiotic Usage:

   - Broad-spectrum antibiotics can indiscriminately target both pathogenic and beneficial bacteria.

   - Prolonged or frequent antibiotic use may lead to persistent alterations in the microbiota composition.

3. Stress and Mental Health:

   - The gut-brain axis plays a crucial role in bidirectional communication between the gut and the central nervous system.

   - Stress-induced changes in gut permeability and motility can contribute to microbial dysbiosis.

4. Infections and Inflammation:

   - Chronic infections and inflammation can alter the local environment, promoting the growth of opportunistic pathogens.

   - Inflammatory mediators can directly impact microbial composition.

Implications of Microbial Dysbiosis in Chronic Conditions

Microbial dysbiosis has been implicated in the pathogenesis of numerous chronic conditions, including but not limited to:

1. Inflammatory Bowel Disease (IBD):

   - Dysbiosis is a hallmark of IBD, with an imbalance in beneficial and pathogenic bacteria.

   - Altered mucosal immunity and impaired barrier function contribute to disease progression.

2. Obesity and Metabolic Syndrome:

- The gut microbiota plays a role in energy extraction from the diet.

- Dysbiosis is associated with metabolic endotoxemia, insulin resistance, and low-grade inflammation.

3. Autoimmune Diseases:

- Dysregulated immune responses can result from altered interactions between the microbiota and the host immune system.

- Rheumatoid arthritis, multiple sclerosis, and systemic lupus erythematosus have all been linked to microbial dysbiosis.

4. Neurological Disorders:

- Growing evidence suggests a connection between gut dysbiosis and neurological conditions.

- Alzheimer's disease, Parkinson's disease, and depression may be influenced by the gut-brain axis.

Therapeutic Approaches to Modulate Microbial Dysbiosis

Addressing microbial dysbiosis presents a promising avenue for therapeutic intervention in chronic conditions. Potential strategies include:

1. Probiotics and Prebiotics:

- Probiotics introduce beneficial bacteria to the gut, promoting a healthy microbial balance.

- Prebiotics provide the substrate for the growth of beneficial microbes.

2. Dietary Modifications:

- Adopting a diet rich in fiber and diverse plant-based foods supports a flourishing microbiota.

- Restricting the intake of processed foods and sugars can mitigate dysbiosis.

3. Fecal Microbiota Transplantation (FMT):

- FMT involves transferring fecal material from a healthy donor to a recipient to restore a balanced microbiota.

- While highly effective for certain conditions, its application requires careful consideration.

4. Antibiotic Stewardship:

- Judicious use of antibiotics, including targeted and narrow-spectrum agents, helps preserve the diversity of the microbiota.

- Combining antibiotic therapy with probiotics may mitigate dysbiosis-associated side effects.

In conclusion, Microbial dysbiosis stands at the crossroads of chronic disease, influencing the onset, progression, and resolution of various conditions. The intricate interplay between the microbiota and the host is a dynamic and evolving field of research. As we deepen our understanding of the mechanisms driving dysbiosis, novel therapeutic strategies are likely to emerge, offering hope for more targeted and personalized approaches to managing chronic conditions. Continued research efforts are essential to unravel the complexities of microbial dysbiosis and harness its potential for improving human health in the years to come.

CHAPTER FOUR

Immune Dysfunction and Chronic Diseases

The human immune system serves as a crucial defense mechanism, safeguarding the body against pathogens, infections, and other external threats. Its intricate network of cells, tissues, and organs works in harmony to maintain a delicate balance between protection and tolerance. However, when this balance is disrupted, immune dysfunction can arise, potentially leading to the development and progression of chronic diseases. This comprehensive exploration delves into the intricate relationship between immune dysfunction and chronic diseases, shedding light on the underlying mechanisms, contributing factors, and potential therapeutic avenues.

The immune system comprises two main branches: the innate immune system and the adaptive immune system. The innate system acts as the first line of defense, providing immediate, nonspecific protection against a wide range of pathogens. On the other hand, the adaptive immune system orchestrates a highly specific response, adapting to encountered threats and forming immunological memory for future encounters.

Immune Dysfunction: A Prelude to Chronic Diseases

1. Inflammatory Pathways and Chronic Inflammation

One of the hallmarks of immune dysfunction is chronic inflammation, a persistent and maladaptive immune response. Chronic inflammation is implicated in the pathogenesis of various chronic diseases, including cardiovascular diseases, diabetes, and neurodegenerative disorders. The constant activation of immune cells and release of pro-inflammatory mediators contribute to tissue damage and dysfunction.

2. Autoimmunity: The Immune System Turned Against Itself

Autoimmune diseases occur when the immune system mistakenly targets and attacks the body's own tissues. Rheumatoid arthritis, lupus, and multiple sclerosis are examples of autoimmune conditions where immune dysfunction leads to chronic inflammation and tissue destruction. Genetic predisposition, environmental factors, and molecular mimicry are among the factors contributing to the development of autoimmune diseases.

3. Immunodeficiency and Increased Susceptibility

Immunodeficiency disorders compromise the body's ability to defend against infections. In conditions such as HIV/AIDS or primary immunodeficiency syndromes, the immune system is weakened, leading to recurrent and severe infections. The prolonged immune compromise in these cases may contribute to the development of chronic diseases.

4. The Gut-Immune Axis: Microbiota and Beyond

The gut plays a pivotal role in immune function, hosting a vast community of microorganisms collectively known as the microbiota. Disruptions in the balance of this complex ecosystem can trigger immune dysfunction. Emerging research suggests that alterations in the gut microbiota may contribute to the development of chronic inflammatory conditions, such as inflammatory bowel disease and metabolic disorders.

Factors Contributing to Immune Dysfunction

1. Genetic Predisposition and Immunogenetics

Genetic factors play a significant role in shaping an individual's immune response. Variations in genes involved in immune regulation and signaling pathways can contribute to susceptibility to immune dysfunction and chronic diseases. Understanding immunogenetics is crucial for unraveling the complex interplay between genetics and the immune system.

2. Environmental Triggers and Exposures

Environmental factors, including exposure to pollutants, toxins, and infectious agents, can modulate immune function. Chronic exposure to environmental stressors may lead to immune dysregulation, increasing the risk of chronic diseases. Investigating the impact of environmental triggers on immune health is essential for developing strategies to mitigate their effects.

3. Lifestyle Factors: Diet, Exercise, and Sleep

Lifestyle choices significantly influence immune function. A balanced diet, regular exercise, and adequate sleep contribute to a well-functioning immune system. Conversely, poor nutrition, sedentary behavior, and sleep deprivation can impair immune responses, creating a conducive environment for the development of chronic diseases.

4. Psychosocial Factors: Stress and Mental Health

The intricate connection between the mind and the immune system is evident in the impact of psychosocial factors on immune function. Chronic stress, anxiety, and depression can dysregulate immune responses, promoting inflammation and contributing to the development of chronic diseases. Exploring the psychoneuroimmunology of immune dysfunction unveils the complex interplay between mental health and immune function.

Clinical Implications and Therapeutic Approaches

1. Immunomodulatory Therapies

Novel therapeutic approaches aim to modulate the immune system to restore balance and alleviate chronic inflammatory conditions. Immunomodulatory drugs, such as biologics and small molecules, target specific components of the immune response. Precision medicine, guided by advances in immunology, enables tailored therapies that address the underlying immune dysfunction in various chronic diseases.

2. The Role of Vaccines in Immune Health

Vaccines play a crucial role in priming the immune system and providing protection against infectious agents. Ongoing research explores the potential of vaccines not only in preventing infections but also in modulating immune responses and potentially preventing or ameliorating chronic diseases. Harnessing the power of vaccination may offer innovative strategies for managing immune dysfunction.

3. Integrative Approaches: Mind-Body Medicine

Integrative medicine approaches, combining conventional and complementary therapies, acknowledge the interconnectedness of physical and mental health. Mind-body practices, such as meditation, yoga, and acupuncture, show promise in modulating immune responses and reducing chronic inflammation. Exploring the integration of these approaches into mainstream healthcare could pave the way for holistic management of immune dysfunction and chronic diseases.

Conclusion

Immune dysfunction stands at the crossroads of numerous chronic diseases, shaping their initiation, progression, and outcomes. Unraveling the complexities of this relationship requires a multidisciplinary approach, integrating insights from immunology, genetics, environmental science, and behavioral medicine. As our understanding of immune dysfunction deepens, so too does the potential for innovative therapeutic interventions that target the root causes of chronic diseases. By addressing immune dysfunction at its core, the path towards personalized and effective management of chronic conditions becomes increasingly tangible, offering hope for improved health outcomes and a better quality of life.

Strategies for Modulating the Immune Response

The immune system is a complex network of cells, tissues, and organs that work together to defend the body against pathogens and maintain homeostasis. However, dysregulation of the immune response can lead to various disorders, ranging from autoimmune diseases to immunodeficiency. The ability to modulate the immune response is a critical aspect of medical research and therapeutic development. This comprehensive exploration delves into the diverse strategies employed to modulate the immune system, examining both conventional and cutting-edge approaches.

1. Immunomodulation: An Overview

Immunomodulation refers to the process of altering the immune response to achieve a desired outcome. This can involve either enhancing or suppressing immune activity, depending on the context. The intricate balance of the immune system is essential for maintaining health, and interventions aimed at modulating this balance hold significant therapeutic potential.

2. Immunosuppressive Therapies

Immunomodulation often involves suppressing the immune response, particularly in conditions where the immune system is overactive. Common strategies include:

- Corticosteroids:

Corticosteroids, such as prednisone, are potent anti-inflammatory agents that suppress immune responses. They are widely used to manage autoimmune diseases and control inflammation.

- Immunosuppressive Drugs:

Medications like methotrexate and cyclosporine inhibit the immune system's activity, making them valuable in the treatment of autoimmune disorders and prevention of organ transplant rejection.

- Monoclonal Antibodies:

Monoclonal antibodies, such as rituximab and infliximab, target specific components of the immune system to modulate its activity. These biologics have revolutionized the treatment of conditions like rheumatoid arthritis and inflammatory bowel disease.

3. Immunostimulatory Approaches

Conversely, there are situations where enhancing the immune response is crucial. Immunostimulatory strategies aim to boost the body's defenses against infections or cancer. Key approaches include:

- Vaccines:

Vaccines are among the most effective and widely used immunostimulatory interventions. They train the immune system to recognize and mount a response against specific pathogens, providing protection against future infections.

- Interferons:

Interferons are signaling proteins that play a central role in antiviral defense. Synthetic interferons are used therapeutically to boost the immune response in conditions like hepatitis and certain cancers.

- Cytokine Therapy:

Administering cytokines, such as interleukins and interferons, can stimulate immune cells. This approach is employed in cancer treatment, enhancing the body's ability to target and destroy malignant cells.

4. Biological Therapies and Targeted Immunomodulation

Advancements in biotechnology have led to the development of targeted immunomodulatory therapies that focus on specific molecules or pathways involved in immune responses. This precision allows for more tailored interventions with potentially fewer side effects. Examples include:

- Checkpoint Inhibitors:

Checkpoint inhibitors, like pembrolizumab and nivolumab, block inhibitory signals in the immune system, enabling T cells to recognize and attack cancer cells. This breakthrough has revolutionized cancer immunotherapy.

- Janus Kinase (JAK) Inhibitors:

JAK inhibitors, such as tofacitinib, modulate immune responses by targeting the Janus kinase pathway. They find application in autoimmune diseases like rheumatoid arthritis.

- Gene Editing Technologies:

Emerging technologies like CRISPR-Cas9 offer the potential to directly modify genes involved in immune responses. While still in the early stages of development, gene editing holds promise for precise immunomodulation.

5. Nutritional Immunomodulation

Diet plays a pivotal role in shaping the immune system. Certain nutrients have been identified for their immunomodulatory properties, and dietary interventions can influence immune function. Key considerations include:

- Vitamins and Minerals:

Micronutrients such as vitamin C, vitamin D, and zinc are essential for immune function. Supplementation or dietary adjustments may be considered to support immune health.

- Probiotics and Prebiotics:

The gut microbiota plays a crucial role in immune regulation. Probiotics (beneficial bacteria) and prebiotics (substrates for beneficial bacteria) contribute to a balanced immune response.

- Anti-Inflammatory Diets:

Diets rich in anti-inflammatory foods, such as omega-3 fatty acids from fish oil and polyphenols from fruits and vegetables, can help modulate immune responses and reduce inflammation.

6. Environmental Factors and Lifestyle Modifications

Beyond medications and dietary interventions, environmental factors and lifestyle choices significantly impact immune function. Key considerations include:

- Exercise:

Regular physical activity is associated with enhanced immune function. Exercise contributes to improved circulation of immune cells and the release of endorphins, promoting overall health.

- Sleep:

Adequate sleep is crucial for immune health. Sleep deprivation can impair immune function, making individuals more susceptible to infections.

- Stress Management:

Chronic stress can have immunosuppressive effects. Stress reduction techniques, such as mindfulness and meditation, may positively influence immune responses.

7. Combination Therapies and Personalized Medicine

Recognizing the complexity of the immune system, researchers are increasingly exploring combination therapies that target multiple aspects of the immune response. Personalized medicine approaches, considering individual variations in immune function and genetic makeup, aim to optimize treatment outcomes.

Modulating the immune response represents a multifaceted challenge with broad implications for human health. From traditional immunosuppressive therapies to cutting-edge biologics and emerging gene editing technologies, the landscape of immunomodulation is continually evolving. Integrating nutritional strategies, considering environmental influences, and embracing personalized medicine further enhance our ability to fine-tune immune responses. As research advances, the potential for innovative approaches to modulate the immune system holds promise for more effective and tailored interventions in the prevention and treatment of immune-related disorders. A comprehensive understanding of these diverse strategies is essential for navigating the complex terrain of immune modulation and improving patient outcomes in the years to come.

CHAPTER FIVE

Technological Advances and Health Consequences

In the ever-evolving landscape of technological progress, the profound impact on human life is undeniable. From the advent of the internet to the proliferation of smartphones and the rise of artificial intelligence, technological advances have transformed the way we live, work, and interact with the world. While these innovations bring unprecedented convenience and efficiency, they also raise important questions about their consequences on human health. This exploration delves into the intricate relationship between technological advances and health, examining both the positive contributions and potential challenges that emerge in this complex interplay.

The Digital Revolution and Connectivity

The digital revolution, marked by the widespread adoption of digital technologies, has ushered in an era of unprecedented connectivity. The internet, a cornerstone of this revolution, has become an integral part of daily life, enabling instant communication, access to information, and global connectivity. Social media platforms, e-commerce, and online services have reshaped the way people connect, share, and conduct business. While these advancements have undoubtedly enhanced efficiency and communication, they also introduce new dynamics that can influence mental and physical well-being.

The rise of social media platforms has redefined the way individuals interact and share experiences. While these platforms offer opportunities for connection and community building, they also present challenges to mental health. The curated nature of social media can contribute to feelings of inadequacy, as individuals compare their lives to carefully crafted online representations. The constant exposure to curated images and narratives may impact self-esteem, fueling anxiety and depression in some individuals.

Moreover, the addictive nature of social media, designed to capture and maintain user attention, raises concerns about excessive screen time. Prolonged use of digital devices, particularly for social media engagement, has been associated with sleep disturbances, eye strain, and sedentary behavior—all of which can have implications for physical and mental health.

Recognizing the potential impact of excessive technology use on well-being, the concept of "digital detox" has gained traction. Digital detox refers to intentional periods of disconnecting from digital devices to promote mental and emotional well-being. This may involve designated time away from screens, engaging in outdoor activities, and fostering face-to-face interactions.

Practicing mindful technology use is another approach that emphasizes conscious and intentional engagement with digital devices. Setting boundaries, such as turning off notifications and establishing screen-free zones, can help mitigate the negative effects of constant connectivity. Cultivating a healthy relationship with technology involves balancing its benefits with intentional efforts to disconnect and engage in activities that promote overall well-being.

Sedentary Lifestyles and Physical Health

The convenience afforded by technological advances has, in some instances, contributed to sedentary lifestyles. Automation, online services, and the prevalence of desk-based jobs have reduced the need for physical activity in daily routines. While technology has brought efficiency and convenience, the shift towards more sedentary lifestyles raises concerns about its impact on physical health.

A sedentary lifestyle is a significant risk factor for various chronic conditions, including obesity, cardiovascular diseases, and metabolic disorders. Lack of regular physical activity contributes to weight gain, impaired metabolic health, and an increased risk of cardiovascular events. The mechanization of tasks that once required physical effort has led to a decline in overall physical activity levels, contributing to the global rise in non-communicable diseases.

The integration of technology into daily life also extends to entertainment, with screen-based activities replacing outdoor play and recreational sports. The seductive allure of video games, streaming services, and online content can contribute to prolonged periods of inactivity, particularly among children and adolescents. Addressing the health consequences of sedentary behavior requires a multifaceted approach that combines awareness, education, and initiatives promoting physical activity.

Counteracting the trend of sedentary lifestyles, wearable technology has emerged as a tool for health monitoring and physical activity promotion. Fitness trackers, smartwatches, and other wearables provide real-time data on steps taken, heart rate, and sleep patterns. These devices offer individuals insights into their activity levels and encourage goal-setting for physical fitness.

The integration of technology into health and wellness extends beyond wearables to include mobile applications and online platforms that provide guided workouts, nutrition tracking, and mental health support. The gamification of fitness, where users engage in challenges and earn rewards for meeting activity goals, adds an element of fun and motivation to physical exercise. As technology continues to evolve, the potential for innovative solutions to promote physical activity and overall health remains promising.

The Impact of Screen Time on Sleep

The prevalence of digital devices has reshaped not only daily routines but also sleep patterns. The use of screens, particularly in the evening, can interfere with the body's natural circadian rhythm and melatonin production. Blue light emitted by screens suppresses melatonin, a hormone that regulates sleep-wake cycles, making it more challenging to fall asleep.

Sleep deprivation, often linked to excessive screen time and late-night device use, has far-reaching consequences for health. Inadequate sleep is associated with an increased risk of obesity, diabetes, cardiovascular diseases, and impaired cognitive function. The constant connectivity facilitated by smartphones and the expectation of immediate responses to messages contribute to disrupted sleep patterns and the blurring of boundaries between work and personal life.

Addressing the impact of screen time on sleep involves adopting sleep hygiene practices. Creating a sleep-friendly environment, establishing a consistent sleep schedule, and implementing digital curfews can help mitigate the negative effects of screen-related sleep disturbances. Educating individuals, especially adolescents who may be more susceptible to sleep disruptions from screen use, about the importance of sleep for overall health is a crucial component of preventive efforts.

Technology and Mental Health: The Double-Edged Sword

While technology has brought unprecedented access to information and communication, its influence on mental health is complex and multifaceted. The digital age has ushered in new challenges and opportunities, with the potential to both support and strain mental well-being.

The abundance of information available online, while empowering, can also lead to information overload. Constant exposure to a barrage of news, notifications, and online content can overwhelm the cognitive capacity to process information. The phenomenon of "doomscrolling," where individuals compulsively scroll through negative news or social media content, contributes to heightened stress levels and anxiety.

Moreover, the rise of misinformation and the rapid dissemination of unverified content pose challenges to mental health. Navigating an online landscape filled with conflicting information requires critical thinking skills and media literacy. The ability to discern credible sources from misinformation is crucial for maintaining mental well-being in the digital age.

Technology has transformed the way people connect and communicate, offering new avenues for social interaction. However, the quality of online social interactions and their impact on mental health warrant careful consideration. While online platforms facilitate connection with friends and communities, they may also contribute to feelings of social isolation and loneliness.

The paradox of social media lies in its ability to connect individuals across distances while potentially eroding the depth of in-person relationships. The curated nature of online interactions, where individuals often showcase highlights rather than authentic experiences, can contribute to a sense of social comparison and the perception of inadequacy.

The digital realm introduces new challenges related to cyberbullying and online harassment, particularly among adolescents. The anonymity afforded by online platforms can embolden individuals to engage in harmful behavior. Cyberbullying, characterized by the use of digital platforms to intimidate, threaten, or harass others, has been linked to adverse mental health outcomes, including depression and anxiety.

Addressing the mental health consequences of online interactions involves fostering digital resilience and promoting positive online behavior. Initiatives aimed at preventing cyberbullying, educating individuals about responsible online conduct, and providing resources for mental health support contribute to creating a safer and more supportive digital environment.

Artificial Intelligence in Healthcare: Opportunities and Ethical Considerations

The integration of artificial intelligence (AI) into healthcare holds immense promise for improving diagnostics, treatment outcomes, and patient care. AI algorithms can analyze vast datasets, identify patterns, and assist healthcare professionals in making more accurate and timely decisions. While the potential benefits of AI in healthcare are significant, ethical considerations and the responsible use of technology are paramount.

AI-powered diagnostic tools have demonstrated remarkable accuracy in identifying medical conditions from medical imaging, pathology slides, and other diagnostic modalities. The ability of AI algorithms to process and analyze complex data sets enables earlier detection of diseases, leading to timely interventions and improved patient outcomes.

In personalized medicine, AI plays a crucial role in analyzing genetic data to identify individualized treatment approaches. By considering an individual's genetic makeup, lifestyle factors, and medical history, AI contributes to tailoring treatment plans that optimize efficacy and minimize potential side effects.

The ethical use of AI in healthcare requires careful consideration of issues related to bias, transparency, and patient privacy. AI algorithms trained on biased datasets may perpetuate and even exacerbate existing healthcare disparities. Ensuring diversity and representativeness in training datasets is essential to prevent algorithmic bias and promote equitable healthcare outcomes.

Transparency in AI decision-making is another ethical consideration. Understanding how AI algorithms arrive at diagnostic or treatment recommendations is crucial for building trust between healthcare professionals, patients, and technology developers. Striking a balance between the complexity of AI algorithms and the need for transparency is an ongoing challenge in the ethical deployment of AI in healthcare.

Patient privacy, a cornerstone of healthcare ethics, becomes increasingly complex in the era of AI. The vast amounts of data required for training AI models, including sensitive health information, raise concerns about data security and the potential for unauthorized access. Robust data

governance frameworks, encryption protocols, and informed consent processes are integral to upholding patient privacy in the age of AI.

The Role of Telemedicine in Healthcare Accessibility

Telemedicine, facilitated by advancements in communication technology, has emerged as a transformative force in healthcare delivery. The ability to connect with healthcare providers remotely has expanded access to medical consultations, especially in underserved and rural areas. While telemedicine offers unparalleled convenience, its widespread adoption also raises considerations related to quality of care, privacy, and the digital divide.

Telemedicine addresses barriers to healthcare access by allowing individuals to consult with healthcare providers from the comfort of their homes. This is particularly beneficial for individuals with mobility issues, those residing in remote areas, and patients with chronic conditions who require ongoing monitoring. The ability to access medical advice through video calls, chat platforms, and remote monitoring devices enhances healthcare accessibility and reduces the need for physical travel.

Ensuring the quality of care in telemedicine involves considerations such as accurate diagnosis, appropriate treatment recommendations, and effective communication between healthcare providers and patients. Digital health literacy, the ability to navigate and understand digital health information and platforms, becomes crucial for patients engaging in telemedicine. Educating individuals about the use of telemedicine, privacy safeguards, and the appropriate channels for seeking medical advice contributes to informed decision-making in the digital healthcare landscape.

While telemedicine offers benefits in terms of accessibility, the digital divide remains a significant challenge. Disparities in access to high-speed internet, digital devices, and technological literacy can limit the reach of telemedicine services. Bridging the digital divide requires comprehensive strategies that address infrastructure gaps, provide digital education, and ensure equitable access to telemedicine resources.

Environmental Impacts of Technology

The rapid pace of technological advancement comes with environmental consequences that warrant attention. The production, use, and disposal of electronic devices contribute to electronic waste (e-waste), a complex environmental challenge. Proper management of e-waste is essential to mitigate environmental pollution and minimize the health risks associated with hazardous materials present in electronic devices.

Electronic devices, such as smartphones, computers, and electronic appliances, contain materials such as lead, mercury, and brominated flame retardants. Improper disposal of e-waste, including burning or landfilling, releases these hazardous substances into the environment. The

contamination of soil, air, and water with toxic elements poses health risks to communities living in proximity to e-waste disposal sites.

Addressing the environmental impacts of technology involves adopting sustainable practices in the design, manufacturing, and disposal of electronic devices. Recycling initiatives, proper e-waste management systems, and regulations that promote eco-friendly product design contribute to minimizing the ecological footprint of technological advancements.

Balancing Innovation with Ethical Considerations

As society continues to embrace technological advances, finding a balance between innovation and ethical considerations becomes imperative. Responsible technology development requires a thoughtful approach that prioritizes human well-being, equity, and environmental sustainability. Ethical frameworks, regulations, and public discourse play pivotal roles in shaping the trajectory of technological progress.

Incorporating ethical considerations into the design and development of technology is fundamental to ensuring positive outcomes for users. User-centric design, which prioritizes the well-being and autonomy of individuals, involves considerations such as privacy protections, transparent algorithms, and user empowerment. Ethical design practices contribute to creating technology that aligns with human values and promotes positive interactions.

Regulatory frameworks play a crucial role in guiding the ethical use of technology. Governments and regulatory bodies are tasked with developing and enforcing policies that address issues such as data privacy, algorithmic accountability, and the ethical deployment of emerging technologies. Balancing the need for innovation with ethical safeguards requires collaboration between policymakers, technology developers, and the broader public.

Engaging the public in discussions about the ethical implications of technology is essential for informed decision-making. Public discourse creates awareness, encourages critical thinking, and holds stakeholders accountable. Educational initiatives that promote digital literacy, media literacy, and ethical considerations in technology use contribute to a more informed and empowered society.

Conclusion: Navigating the Intersection of Technology and Health

The complex interplay between technological advances and health underscores the need for a holistic and proactive approach. While technology brings undeniable benefits in terms of connectivity, healthcare accessibility, and information dissemination, it also introduces challenges that require careful consideration. Ethical frameworks, responsible innovation, and informed decision-making serve as pillars for navigating the intersection of technology and health.

As society continues to harness the power of technology, the quest for balance remains ongoing. Embracing the positive contributions of technological advances while addressing potential pitfalls

requires collaboration across disciplines, industries, and communities. By fostering a collective commitment to ethical technology use, prioritizing human well-being, and safeguarding the environment, society can navigate the complex landscape of technological progress with a focus on creating a future where innovation aligns harmoniously with health and societal values.

Urbanization, Stress, and Their Toll on Well-being

The rapid pace of urbanization in the modern era has transformed the global landscape, with more people than ever before residing in cities. While urban environments offer economic opportunities, cultural richness, and access to diverse amenities, they also bring forth a unique set of challenges that can impact individual well-being. One notable consequence of urban living is the heightened prevalence of stressors, stemming from factors such as overcrowding, noise pollution, and the fast-paced lifestyle characteristic of cities. This exploration delves into the complex interplay between urbanization, stress, and their repercussions on overall well-being.

Urbanization, the process of population concentration in cities and the growth of urban areas, is a defining feature of contemporary societal development. Over the past century, the global population has undergone a significant shift from predominantly rural to predominantly urban. This urban transition has been fueled by factors such as industrialization, technological advancements, and migration patterns, drawing individuals to urban centers in search of employment, education, and improved living standards.

Cities serve as hubs of economic activity, providing job opportunities and fostering innovation. The concentration of businesses, educational institutions, and cultural establishments in urban areas attracts individuals seeking a spectrum of experiences. The diversity of urban populations contributes to a rich tapestry of cultures, ideas, and perspectives. The promise of economic prosperity and cultural vibrancy propels the ongoing trend of urbanization, shaping the demographic landscape of nations around the world.

Urbanization is often accompanied by extensive infrastructure development, including transportation networks, communication systems, and public services. Skyscrapers, bridges, and

modern amenities characterize urban landscapes, symbolizing progress and connectivity. The allure of improved infrastructure, coupled with the potential for social and economic mobility, continues to draw individuals from rural areas to cities in pursuit of a better quality of life.

The Stressors of Urban Living

While urbanization brings about numerous benefits, it also exposes individuals to a myriad of stressors inherent to city life. The unique challenges posed by urban environments can have profound effects on mental and physical well-being. Understanding the nature of these stressors is crucial for developing strategies to mitigate their impact and foster resilience in urban populations.

One of the primary stressors associated with urban living is overcrowding. The high population density in cities often results in limited living space, cramped public transportation, and congested public areas. Overcrowding can evoke feelings of claustrophobia, exacerbate social tensions, and contribute to a sense of anonymity that may impact social cohesion. The constant proximity to large numbers of people can be emotionally draining, leading to increased stress levels.

Urban environments are characterized by a cacophony of sounds—traffic, construction, sirens, and the hum of daily activities. The pervasive nature of noise in cities contributes to a phenomenon known as noise pollution. Chronic exposure to elevated noise levels has been linked to a range of health issues, including increased stress, sleep disturbances, and heightened risk of cardiovascular problems. The continuous barrage of urban noise can elevate stress hormone levels, leading to a state of chronic arousal that negatively affects both mental and physical health.

Cities are synonymous with a fast-paced lifestyle, characterized by hectic schedules, demanding work hours, and a constant sense of time pressure. The pressure to keep up with the rapid pace of urban life can contribute to heightened stress levels and burnout. The pursuit of career goals, academic achievements, and social engagements in the urban milieu can lead to a perpetual sense of urgency, impacting mental well-being and contributing to conditions such as anxiety and depression.

Urban environments often grapple with elevated levels of air pollution, resulting from vehicular emissions, industrial activities, and other sources. Exposure to air pollutants has been linked to respiratory problems, cardiovascular diseases, and adverse neurological effects. Additionally, the urban heat island effect, where cities experience higher temperatures than surrounding rural areas, can exacerbate the impact of heatwaves, posing risks to vulnerable populations and increasing the overall stress on urban ecosystems.

The Psychological Impact of Urban Stress

The psychological impact of urban stressors extends beyond immediate feelings of discomfort, influencing mental health outcomes and overall well-being. The chronic exposure to stress in urban environments can contribute to the development or exacerbation of mental health conditions,

presenting a multifaceted challenge that requires comprehensive understanding and targeted interventions.

Epidemiological studies have consistently highlighted the association between urban living and an increased prevalence of mental health disorders. Conditions such as anxiety disorders, depression, and substance abuse have been linked to the stressors inherent in urban environments. The complex interplay of socio-economic factors, environmental stressors, and individual vulnerabilities contributes to the heightened risk of mental health challenges in urban populations.

Chronic stress, a common outcome of prolonged exposure to urban stressors, can have profound implications for physical health. The stress response, characterized by the release of stress hormones such as cortisol, is designed to mobilize the body's resources to cope with immediate threats. However, when stress becomes chronic, the continuous activation of the stress response can contribute to systemic inflammation, immune dysfunction, and an increased risk of chronic diseases such as cardiovascular disorders, diabetes, and autoimmune conditions.

Coping Mechanisms and Resilience in Urban Environments

While urban living poses unique challenges to well-being, individuals and communities often develop coping mechanisms and resilience strategies to navigate the complexities of city life. Understanding these adaptive processes is essential for promoting mental health and fostering a sense of community in urban environments.

Social support networks play a crucial role in mitigating the impact of urban stress. The formation of close-knit communities, whether within neighborhoods, workplaces, or cultural groups, provides a buffer against the isolating effects of urban living. Social connections offer emotional support, a sense of belonging, and opportunities for collective problem-solving, enhancing individuals' ability to cope with stressors.

The availability of green spaces and access to nature within urban settings can contribute significantly to well-being. Urban planning that prioritizes parks, gardens, and recreational areas provides residents with opportunities to engage in outdoor activities, connect with nature, and experience relaxation. Exposure to green spaces has been associated with improved mental health outcomes, stress reduction, and enhanced overall life satisfaction.

Practices such as mindfulness meditation, yoga, and stress reduction techniques offer individuals tools to manage and alleviate urban stress. Mindfulness, characterized by present-moment awareness and non-judgmental attention, has been shown to reduce stress levels, improve mental clarity, and enhance emotional well-being. Integrating mindfulness practices into daily routines can empower individuals to cultivate resilience in the face of urban challenges.

Urban planning and design play pivotal roles in shaping the well-being of city residents. Thoughtful urban design that prioritizes pedestrian-friendly spaces, efficient public transportation, and aesthetically pleasing environments contributes to a positive urban experience. Creating

walkable neighborhoods, incorporating green infrastructure, and addressing issues such as traffic congestion and air quality are integral components of designing cities that promote well-being.

Addressing Urban Stress at the Policy Level

Effectively addressing urban stress requires a multi-faceted approach that encompasses policy interventions, community engagement, and public health initiatives. Policymakers play a central role in shaping the urban landscape and implementing strategies to enhance the well-being of residents.

Incorporating well-being considerations into urban planning and design guidelines is essential for creating cities that prioritize the health of residents. Designing spaces that promote physical activity, offer access to greenery, and minimize noise pollution contributes to a more conducive urban environment. Urban planners can collaborate with architects, environmental scientists, and public health experts to integrate well-being principles into the fabric of urban development.

Transportation policies play a critical role in addressing urban stressors related to traffic congestion and air pollution. Investing in sustainable transportation infrastructure, promoting public transit, and incentivizing non-motorized modes of transportation contribute to reducing the environmental impact of urban mobility. Improving air quality through emissions controls and promoting active transportation options, such as cycling and walking, fosters a healthier urban environment.

Raising awareness about mental health and providing accessible support services are integral components of addressing the mental health challenges associated with urban living. Community-based mental health initiatives, public awareness campaigns, and the integration of mental health services into primary care contribute to reducing the stigma surrounding mental health and facilitating early intervention.

Green urban interventions, such as the creation of urban forests, green roofs, and community gardens, contribute to mitigating the environmental stressors associated with urban living. These interventions enhance biodiversity, improve air quality, and create recreational spaces that promote physical and mental well-being. Collaborative efforts between local governments, environmental organizations, and community groups can drive the implementation of green initiatives at the neighborhood level.

The Future of Urban Well-being

As urbanization continues to shape the global landscape, the quest for urban well-being becomes an increasingly pressing concern. The future of cities lies in the ability to strike a balance between economic growth, technological innovation, and the promotion of human flourishing. Embracing a holistic approach that considers the diverse needs of urban populations and prioritizes sustainability is essential for creating cities where residents thrive.

The concept of smart cities, leveraging technology to enhance urban living, holds promise for addressing some of the challenges associated with urban stress. Technological innovations, such as real-time monitoring of air quality, smart traffic management, and data-driven urban planning, contribute to creating more efficient, sustainable, and livable cities. Integrating technology into urban governance and infrastructure has the potential to enhance the well-being of residents and improve the overall urban experience.

Empowering communities to actively participate in the decision-making processes that shape their urban environment is a key element of fostering well-being. Community engagement initiatives, participatory urban planning, and collaborative projects that address the unique needs of diverse populations contribute to creating inclusive and resilient cities. Recognizing the agency of residents in shaping the future of their communities strengthens the social fabric and enhances overall urban well-being.

Sustainable urban development, encompassing environmentally friendly practices, equitable resource distribution, and social inclusivity, is fundamental to the well-being of current and future urban populations. Balancing economic growth with environmental stewardship, promoting social equity, and ensuring the availability of essential resources contribute to the creation of cities that prioritize the health and happiness of residents.

Urbanization, stress, and their impact on well-being form a complex tapestry that requires careful consideration and intentional interventions. As cities continue to evolve, the pursuit of urban well-being demands a holistic approach that integrates urban planning, public health, community engagement, and technological innovation. By fostering environments that prioritize human flourishing, promote social connection, and address the unique stressors of urban living, society can navigate the urban landscape with a focus on creating cities where individuals not only survive but thrive.

CHAPTER SIX

The Role of Nutrition in Chronic Conditions

Nutrition, the intake of food and its subsequent utilization by the body, is a fundamental aspect of human health. The impact of nutrition extends far beyond fulfilling basic dietary requirements; it plays a pivotal role in preventing, managing, and sometimes even reversing chronic conditions. Chronic diseases, characterized by long durations and often slow progression, include conditions such as cardiovascular diseases, diabetes, obesity, and certain cancers. Understanding the intricate interplay between nutrition and chronic conditions is essential for promoting health, preventing disease, and optimizing overall well-being.

Before delving into the specific relationship between nutrition and chronic conditions, it's crucial to establish the foundational principles of nutrition. Nutrients, the substances obtained from food that the body needs for growth, maintenance, and repair, are classified into macronutrients and micronutrients.

Macronutrients

1. Carbohydrates: The primary source of energy for the body, carbohydrates are broken down into glucose, which serves as a fuel for various cellular processes. Sources of carbohydrates include fruits, vegetables, grains, and legumes.

2. Proteins: Essential for the structure, function, and regulation of the body's tissues and organs, proteins are composed of amino acids. Dietary protein sources include meat, dairy products, legumes, and plant-based proteins.

3. Fats: Fats play a crucial role in energy storage, insulation, and the absorption of fat-soluble vitamins. Healthy fats are found in sources such as avocados, nuts, seeds, and olive oil.

Micronutrients

1. Vitamins: Essential for various physiological processes, vitamins are divided into water-soluble (e.g., vitamin C, B-complex vitamins) and fat-soluble (e.g., vitamins A, D, E, K) categories. Each vitamin plays a specific role in supporting overall health.

2. Minerals: Minerals, such as calcium, iron, magnesium, and zinc, are essential for functions like bone health, oxygen transport, and enzyme activity. These micronutrients are obtained through a diverse and balanced diet.

Nutrition and Chronic Diseases

The link between nutrition and chronic diseases is multifaceted, involving factors such as dietary patterns, nutrient composition, and individual variations in metabolism. Dietary choices influence the risk, development, and management of chronic conditions. Examining the impact of nutrition on specific chronic diseases provides insights into the preventive and therapeutic potential of dietary interventions.

Cardiovascular Diseases

Cardiovascular diseases (CVD), encompassing conditions like coronary artery disease and stroke, are major contributors to global morbidity and mortality. Nutrition plays a crucial role in influencing risk factors associated with CVD, including hypertension, dyslipidemia, and inflammation.

1. Dietary Patterns: The Mediterranean diet, characterized by a high intake of fruits, vegetables, whole grains, fish, and olive oil, has been associated with a lower risk of CVD. This dietary pattern emphasizes unsaturated fats, antioxidants, and anti-inflammatory foods.

2. Omega-3 Fatty Acids: Found in fatty fish, flaxseeds, and walnuts, omega-3 fatty acids contribute to cardiovascular health by reducing inflammation, improving lipid profiles, and supporting arterial function.

3. Fiber: A high-fiber diet, obtained from fruits, vegetables, and whole grains, has been linked to lower cholesterol levels, improved blood glucose control, and a reduced risk of developing CVD.

4. Sodium Restriction: Limiting sodium intake is crucial for managing hypertension, a significant risk factor for CVD. A diet rich in potassium from fruits and vegetables helps counterbalance the effects of sodium.

Diabetes

Diabetes, characterized by elevated blood glucose levels, encompasses type 1 and type 2 diabetes. Nutrition plays a central role in managing blood glucose levels, preventing complications, and improving overall diabetes management.

1. Carbohydrate Management: Monitoring carbohydrate intake is essential for individuals with diabetes. Emphasizing complex carbohydrates, such as whole grains and legumes, and moderating the intake of simple sugars contribute to better glycemic control.

2. Dietary Fiber: Fiber-rich foods, including vegetables, fruits, and whole grains, have benefits for individuals with diabetes. Fiber slows the absorption of glucose, helping to stabilize blood sugar levels.

3. Protein Intake: Including lean protein sources, such as poultry, fish, tofu, and legumes, can contribute to satiety and assist in managing blood glucose levels.

4. Healthy Fats: Choosing heart-healthy fats, such as those found in avocados, nuts, and olive oil, is important for individuals with diabetes to reduce the risk of cardiovascular complications.

Obesity

Obesity, a complex condition involving an excessive accumulation of body fat, is a major risk factor for numerous chronic diseases, including diabetes, CVD, and certain cancers. Nutrition plays a central role in both the prevention and management of obesity.

1. Caloric Balance: Achieving and maintaining a healthy weight involves balancing caloric intake with expenditure. Nutrient-dense, lower-calorie foods contribute to a sustainable and health-promoting diet.

2. Portion Control: Monitoring portion sizes and practicing mindful eating are essential for weight management. Awareness of portion control helps prevent excessive calorie consumption.

3. Nutrient Composition: Beyond calorie counting, the quality of nutrients matters. A diet rich in fruits, vegetables, lean proteins, and whole grains provides essential nutrients while promoting satiety.

4. Physical Activity: Nutrition and physical activity are interconnected in the management of obesity. A balanced diet, coupled with regular exercise, supports weight loss and overall well-being.

Cancer

Nutrition plays a crucial role in influencing cancer risk and progression. Dietary patterns and specific nutrients have been associated with either an increased or decreased risk of certain cancer.

1. Plant-Based Diets: Diets rich in fruits, vegetables, and plant-based foods have been linked to a lower risk of several cancers. Antioxidants and phytochemicals found in plant foods contribute to cellular protection.

2. Limiting Processed Meats: Consumption of processed meats, high in additives and preservatives, has been associated with an increased risk of colorectal cancer. Choosing lean proteins and incorporating plant-based protein sources is advisable.

3. Vitamin D: Adequate vitamin D levels, obtained from sunlight exposure and dietary sources such as fatty fish and fortified foods, are associated with a reduced risk of certain cancers, including breast and colorectal cancer.

4. Antioxidants: Antioxidant-rich foods, such as berries, nuts, and leafy greens, help neutralize free radicals and reduce oxidative stress, contributing to cancer prevention.

Nutrigenomics: Personalized Nutrition

The field of nutrigenomics explores how individual genetic variations influence responses to nutrients and dietary patterns. Personalized nutrition, guided by genetic information, tailors dietary recommendations to an individual's unique genetic profile.

1. Genetic Variations: Certain genetic variations impact how individuals metabolize nutrients, respond to dietary components, and modulate disease risk. Understanding these variations enables personalized dietary recommendations.

2. Nutrient-Gene Interactions: Nutrients can influence gene expression and function. For example, omega-3 fatty acids may modulate inflammation-related genes, showcasing the intricate interplay between nutrition and genetics.

3. Precision Nutrition: Integrating genetic information with dietary guidance allows for precision nutrition, where individuals receive personalized recommendations based on their unique genetic makeup and health goals.

Challenges in Nutritional Approaches

While the impact of nutrition on chronic conditions is evident, several challenges exist in implementing effective nutritional approaches at individual and population levels.

1. Socioeconomic Disparities: Access to nutritious foods and resources for healthy living is not uniform across populations. Socioeconomic factors influence dietary choices, creating disparities in nutritional health.

2. Nutrition Education: Limited nutrition education and awareness contribute to unhealthy dietary habits. Empowering individuals with accurate and accessible nutrition information is crucial for promoting better food choices.

3. Cultural and Dietary Preferences: Cultural influences and individual dietary preferences shape eating habits. Tailoring nutritional guidance to align with diverse cultural contexts enhances the likelihood of successful adoption.

4. Food Environment: The availability and marketing of unhealthy food options contribute to suboptimal dietary choices. Creating supportive food environments through policy interventions can positively influence dietary behaviors.

Future Directions in Nutritional Research

Continued research in nutrition and chronic conditions holds promise for uncovering novel insights and refining dietary recommendations. Emerging areas of interest include:

1. Gut Microbiota: The gut microbiota, comprising trillions of microorganisms in the digestive tract, plays a role in nutrient metabolism and overall health. Research exploring the link between gut microbiota, nutrition, and chronic conditions is ongoing.

2. Nutraceuticals: Nutraceuticals, bioactive compounds found in certain foods or available as supplements, show potential in preventing or managing chronic diseases. Studying the efficacy and safety of nutraceutical interventions is an evolving field.

3. Epigenetics: Epigenetic modifications, alterations in gene expression that do not involve changes to the underlying DNA sequence, are influenced by nutrition. Understanding how nutrition impacts epigenetic mechanisms offers insights into disease prevention.

4. Digital Health and Nutrition Apps: The integration of digital health platforms and nutrition apps provides tools for individuals to monitor and improve their dietary habits. Research on the effectiveness of digital interventions in promoting healthy nutrition is advancing.

Empowering Health Through Nutrition

Nutrition stands as a cornerstone in the intricate web of factors influencing chronic conditions. As research advances and our understanding of the nuanced relationship between nutrition and health deepens, opportunities emerge to harness the preventive and therapeutic potential of dietary interventions. Empowering individuals with knowledge, promoting access to nutritious foods, and addressing systemic challenges are integral components of leveraging nutrition to enhance health, prevent chronic diseases, and foster well-being across diverse populations.

Crafting a Healing Diet: Nourishing the Body, Mind, and Spirit

The concept of a healing diet goes beyond mere sustenance; it embodies the philosophy that food is medicine. Crafting a healing diet involves intentional choices aimed at nourishing not only the body but also the mind and spirit. This holistic approach recognizes the interconnectedness of physical, mental, and emotional well-being. In a world where lifestyles are often fast-paced and stress is pervasive, adopting a healing diet can be a transformative journey toward optimal health. This exploration delves into the principles, components, and potential benefits of crafting a healing diet.

Foundational Principles of a Healing Diet

1. Whole, Nutrient-Dense Foods: At the core of a healing diet are whole, nutrient-dense foods that provide essential vitamins, minerals, and phytonutrients. Emphasizing a colorful array of fruits and vegetables, whole grains, lean proteins, and healthy fats forms the foundation of nutritional excellence.

2. Inflammation Reduction: Chronic inflammation is implicated in various health conditions, from cardiovascular diseases to autoimmune disorders. A healing diet focuses on anti-inflammatory foods, including fatty fish rich in omega-3 fatty acids, turmeric, ginger, and a variety of fruits and vegetables.

3. Balanced Macronutrients: Achieving a balance of macronutrients—carbohydrates, proteins, and fats—is key to sustaining energy levels, promoting satiety, and supporting overall health. The emphasis is on choosing complex carbohydrates, lean proteins, and heart-healthy fats.

4. Mindful Eating Practices: Mindful eating involves cultivating awareness and paying attention to the sensory experience of eating. This includes savoring flavors, appreciating textures, and recognizing hunger and fullness cues. Mindful eating fosters a positive relationship with food and promotes digestive well-being.

5. Hydration: A healing diet recognizes the importance of proper hydration for overall health. Water supports digestion, nutrient absorption, and detoxification processes. Herbal teas and infused water with natural flavors enhance hydration while avoiding sugary beverages.

Components of a Healing Diet

1. Fruits and Vegetables:

 - Colorful Variety: Different colors in fruits and vegetables signify diverse phytonutrients, each offering unique health benefits. Berries, leafy greens, citrus fruits, and cruciferous vegetables contribute to a rich spectrum of nutrients.

 - Fiber-Rich Choices: Fiber supports digestive health, regulates blood sugar levels, and promotes satiety. Whole fruits, vegetables, legumes, and whole grains are excellent sources of dietary fiber.

2. Whole Grains:

 - Ancient Grains: Incorporating ancient grains such as quinoa, farro, and millet provides a nutrient-dense alternative to refined grains. These grains offer a variety of vitamins, minerals, and antioxidants.

3. Lean Proteins:

 - Fatty Fish: Rich in omega-3 fatty acids, fatty fish like salmon, mackerel, and sardines contribute to heart health and may have anti-inflammatory effects.

 - Plant-Based Proteins: Legumes, tofu, tempeh, and a variety of nuts and seeds are plant-based protein sources that offer essential amino acids and plant compounds.

4. Healthy Fats:

 - Avocado: Avocados provide monounsaturated fats, which support heart health and are a rich source of vitamins and minerals.

 - Nuts and Seeds: Almonds, walnuts, chia seeds, and flaxseeds offer a combination of healthy fats, fiber, and micronutrients.

5. Herbs and Spices:

 - Turmeric: Known for its anti-inflammatory properties, turmeric contains curcumin, a bioactive compound with potential health benefits.

 - Ginger: Ginger has anti-nausea and anti-inflammatory effects, contributing to digestive health.

6. Fermented Foods:

 - Yogurt: Probiotics in yogurt promote gut health by supporting the balance of beneficial bacteria in the digestive system.

- Kimchi and Sauerkraut: Fermented vegetables contribute to a healthy gut microbiota, which is linked to various aspects of overall health.

7. Herbal Teas:

- Chamomile: Chamomile tea has calming properties and may promote relaxation, making it a soothing choice for mental well-being.

- Peppermint: Peppermint tea may aid digestion and alleviate symptoms of indigestion.

8. Colorful Berries:

- Antioxidant-Rich Choices: Berries such as blueberries, strawberries, and raspberries are rich in antioxidants, which help combat oxidative stress and inflammation.

Potential Benefits of a Healing Diet

1. Inflammation Reduction:

- Anti-Inflammatory Foods: Consuming foods with anti-inflammatory properties, such as fatty fish, turmeric, and leafy greens, may help reduce chronic inflammation associated with various diseases.

2. Heart Health:

- Omega-3 Fatty Acids: Fatty fish, flaxseeds, and walnuts, rich in omega-3 fatty acids, contribute to cardiovascular health by reducing blood clotting, lowering blood pressure, and improving lipid profiles.

3. Digestive Well-Being:

- Fiber-Rich Foods: A diet abundant in fiber supports digestive health by promoting regular bowel movements, preventing constipation, and nourishing the gut microbiota.

4. Blood Sugar Regulation:

- Complex Carbohydrates: Choosing complex carbohydrates with a low glycemic index helps regulate blood sugar levels, reducing the risk of insulin resistance and type 2 diabetes.

5. Mental Health Support:

- Nutrient-Rich Foods: Nutrient-dense foods provide essential vitamins and minerals that support brain health, potentially influencing mood and cognitive function.

- Omega-3 Fatty Acids: The role of omega-3 fatty acids in brain health is being explored, with some studies suggesting a positive impact on mental well-being.

6. Weight Management:

- Satiety from Nutrient-Dense Foods: Nutrient-dense foods promote satiety, reducing the likelihood of overeating and supporting weight management.

- Balanced Macronutrients: A balanced distribution of macronutrients contributes to sustained energy levels, preventing energy crashes that can lead to unhealthy food choices.

7. Gut Microbiota Diversity:

- Fermented Foods: Incorporating fermented foods contributes to a diverse and balanced gut microbiota, which is associated with various aspects of health, including immune function and metabolism.

Crafting a Healing Diet for Individual Needs

1. Bioindividuality:

- Unique Dietary Requirements: Recognizing bioindividuality acknowledges that each person may have unique dietary needs based on factors such as genetics, metabolism, and health conditions.

- Allergies and Sensitivities: Tailoring a healing diet involves considering individual allergies, intolerances, and sensitivities to specific foods.

2. Intuitive Eating:

- Listening to Body Signals: Intuitive eating involves paying attention to hunger and fullness cues, as well as cravings. It encourages mindful eating and fosters a positive relationship with food.

3. Cultural Considerations:

- Culinary Diversity: Crafting a healing diet takes into account the rich diversity of culinary traditions worldwide. Embracing cultural preferences enhances the sustainability and enjoyment of the chosen dietary approach.

4. Collaboration with Healthcare Professionals:

- Nutritional Guidance: Individuals with specific health conditions or dietary restrictions benefit from collaborating with healthcare professionals, including registered dietitians and nutritionists.

- Medical Conditions: Crafting a healing diet for managing medical conditions requires consideration of specific dietary modifications. Conditions such as celiac disease, irritable bowel syndrome (IBS), and food allergies necessitate tailored dietary approaches.

Challenges and Considerations in Adopting a Healing Diet

1. Accessibility and Affordability:

- Nutrient-Rich Foods: Some nutrient-dense foods may be less accessible or more expensive, posing challenges for individuals with limited access to fresh produce or specialty items.

- Addressing Disparities: Addressing disparities in access to healthy foods is essential for promoting equitable opportunities for individuals to adopt a healing diet.

2. Culinary Skills and Time Constraints:

- Cooking Knowledge: The preparation of whole, nutrient-dense foods may require culinary skills that individuals may need to develop over time.

- Time-Intensive Preparation: The perception that a healing diet is time-consuming may deter some individuals, highlighting the need for education on quick and accessible recipes.

3. Cultural Sensitivity:

- Cultural Perspectives: Cultural preferences and dietary traditions vary widely. A one-size-fits-all approach may not be suitable, emphasizing the importance of culturally sensitive dietary guidance.

- Respecting Traditions: Crafting a healing diet involves respecting and integrating cultural traditions, ensuring that individuals can embrace dietary changes while staying connected to their heritage.

4. Psychosocial Factors:

- Emotional Connections to Food: Addressing emotional connections to food is crucial, as individuals may use food as a coping mechanism for stress, sadness, or other emotions.

- Social Aspects of Eating: Social dynamics and cultural norms surrounding food play a role in dietary choices. Strategies for navigating social situations while adhering to a healing diet are important for long-term success.

Future Directions in Healing Diet Research

1. Personalized Nutrition:

  - Nutrigenomics: Advancements in nutrigenomics, the study of how individual genetics influence responses to nutrients, hold promise for personalized nutrition approaches.

  - Precision Diets: Tailoring dietary recommendations based on an individual's genetic makeup, metabolic profile, and health goals is an emerging area of research.

2. Gut Microbiota and Health:

  - Microbiome Research: Further exploration of the gut microbiota and its role in health is underway. Understanding how dietary choices influence the microbiome contributes to personalized dietary recommendations.

3. Food-Brain Connection:

  - Neuro-nutrition: Investigating the food-brain connection and how specific nutrients impact cognitive function, mood, and mental well-being is an evolving area of interest.

4. Community-Based Approaches:

  - Public Health Initiatives: Community-based initiatives that promote access to healthy foods, provide nutrition education, and address systemic factors contribute to improved public health outcomes.

  - Collaboration with Communities: Collaborative efforts involving healthcare professionals, community leaders, and individuals enhance the effectiveness of community-based approaches.

A Holistic Approach to Well-Being

Crafting a healing diet is a journey that extends beyond the plate, embracing the interconnected nature of body, mind, and spirit. By intentionally choosing foods that nourish and support overall health, individuals can embark on a transformative path toward well-being. Recognizing the diversity of nutritional needs, cultural influences, and individual preferences is integral to making a healing diet accessible and sustainable for diverse populations. As research continues to unravel the intricate connections between nutrition and health, the potential for personalized and community-based approaches holds the promise of empowering individuals to thrive on their unique paths to well-being.

CHAPTER SEVEN

Integrative Approaches to Treatment in Chronic Illness

Chronic illnesses, characterized by prolonged durations and often slow progression, pose significant challenges to individuals and healthcare systems worldwide. The conventional model of healthcare, centered around pharmacological interventions and symptom management, is evolving to incorporate integrative approaches that embrace a more holistic paradigm. Integrative medicine, an approach that combines conventional medical treatments with complementary and alternative therapies, seeks to address the complex interplay of physical, mental, and emotional factors inherent in chronic conditions. This exploration delves into the principles, modalities, and potential benefits of integrative approaches to treatment in chronic illness.

Principles of Integrative Medicine

1. Patient-Centered Care:

- Holistic Assessment: Integrative medicine emphasizes a comprehensive assessment that considers not only physical symptoms but also the individual's mental, emotional, and spiritual well-being.

- Shared Decision-Making: Collaborative decision-making between healthcare providers and patients fosters a sense of empowerment and ensures that treatment plans align with the patient's values and preferences.

2. Mind-Body Connection:

- Psychoneuroimmunology: The field of psychoneuroimmunology explores the bidirectional communication between the nervous, endocrine, and immune systems. Integrative approaches recognize the influence of mental and emotional states on physical health.

- Mindfulness and Stress Reduction: Practices such as mindfulness meditation, yoga, and relaxation techniques are integral components of integrative care, addressing the impact of stress on chronic conditions.

3. Personalized Medicine:

- Individual Variability: Recognizing that individuals respond differently to treatments, integrative medicine tailors interventions based on the unique characteristics of each patient.

- Genomic Medicine: Advances in genomics contribute to personalized medicine by identifying genetic factors that influence responses to medications and susceptibility to certain conditions.

4. Promotion of Health and Prevention:

- Lifestyle Modifications: Integrative medicine places a strong emphasis on lifestyle interventions, including dietary changes, physical activity, and stress management, as preventive measures against the progression of chronic diseases.

- Patient Education: Empowering patients with knowledge about their conditions and encouraging proactive health behaviors are central to integrative care.

Modalities of Integrative Medicine

1. Nutritional Medicine:

- Therapeutic Diets: Integrative healthcare providers may recommend specific diets tailored to address the nutritional needs of individuals with chronic conditions. For example, anti-inflammatory diets for conditions associated with systemic inflammation.

- Nutraceuticals: The use of nutraceuticals, including vitamins, minerals, and herbal supplements, is integrated into treatment plans to support overall health and address specific nutritional deficiencies.

2. Mind-Body Therapies:

- Mindfulness-Based Stress Reduction (MBSR): MBSR programs incorporate mindfulness meditation, yoga, and awareness techniques to reduce stress and improve psychological well-being in individuals with chronic illnesses.

- Cognitive-Behavioral Therapy (CBT): CBT, a form of psychotherapy, addresses the relationship between thoughts, feelings, and behaviors. It is utilized to manage symptoms and improve coping mechanisms.

3. Acupuncture and Traditional Chinese Medicine (TCM):

- Acupuncture: Acupuncture involves the insertion of thin needles into specific points on the body to promote the flow of energy (Qi) and restore balance. It is used to alleviate pain, manage symptoms, and enhance overall well-being.

- Herbal Medicine: Integrative practitioners may incorporate herbal remedies based on TCM principles to address imbalances and support the body's natural healing processes.

4. Physical Therapies:

- Massage Therapy: Massage is utilized to reduce muscle tension, improve circulation, and promote relaxation. It is often integrated into treatment plans for conditions involving musculoskeletal issues.

- Exercise Therapy: Tailored exercise programs, including aerobic and strength training, are prescribed to enhance physical function, reduce fatigue, and improve quality of life in individuals with chronic illnesses.

5. Energy Therapies:

- Reiki: Reiki is a form of energy healing that involves the channeling of universal energy to promote balance and facilitate the body's natural healing processes. It is used to address energy imbalances and promote relaxation.

- Biofield Therapies: Practices such as therapeutic touch and healing touch involve the manipulation of the body's energy field to promote physical and emotional well-being.

6. Chiropractic Care:

- Spinal Adjustments: Chiropractic adjustments focus on the alignment of the spine to promote optimal nervous system function. Chiropractic care is often sought for musculoskeletal conditions and pain management.

7. Mind-Body Movement Practices:

- Yoga: Yoga integrates physical postures, breathwork, and meditation to enhance flexibility, strength, and mental clarity. It is utilized as a therapeutic modality for various chronic conditions.

- Tai Chi: Tai Chi, an ancient Chinese martial art, combines gentle movements with deep breathing and meditation. It is beneficial for improving balance, reducing stress, and enhancing overall well-being.

Benefits of Integrative Approaches in Chronic Illness

1. Symptom Management:

- Pain Relief: Integrative modalities such as acupuncture, massage, and chiropractic care contribute to pain relief and improved musculoskeletal function.

- Stress Reduction: Mind-body therapies, including mindfulness and relaxation techniques, reduce stress levels, positively impacting mental and emotional well-being.

2. Quality of Life Improvement:

- Enhanced Physical Function: Physical therapies and exercise interventions enhance mobility, reduce fatigue, and contribute to an improved quality of life for individuals with chronic illnesses.

- Emotional Well-Being: Integrative approaches address the emotional aspects of chronic conditions, promoting mental well-being and a positive outlook on life.

3. Supportive Cancer Care:

- Complementary Therapies: Integrative approaches are often integrated into cancer care to support symptom management, alleviate treatment side effects, and improve the overall quality of life for cancer patients.

- Mind-Body Support: Mind-body practices contribute to the emotional and psychological well-being of individuals undergoing cancer treatment, aiding in coping and resilience.

4. Chronic Disease Prevention:

- Lifestyle Modifications: Integrative medicine promotes lifestyle changes, including dietary modifications and stress reduction, as preventive measures against the progression of chronic diseases.

- Health Promotion: Integrative care focuses on promoting overall health and well-being, addressing factors that contribute to chronic disease development.

5. Individual Empowerment:

- Patient-Centered Approach: Integrative care empowers individuals by involving them in the decision-making process and providing education about their conditions and treatment options.

- Self-Management: Integrative approaches often include strategies for self-management, allowing individuals to actively participate in their care and make informed choices.

Challenges and Considerations in Integrative Medicine

1. Integration with Conventional Care:

   - Communication among Providers: Effective communication and collaboration between integrative practitioners and conventional healthcare providers are crucial to ensure cohesive and safe patient care.

   - Evidence-Based Practices: The integration of evidence-based complementary therapies into conventional care requires ongoing research and a commitment to maintaining high standards of safety and efficacy.

2. Insurance Coverage:

   - Reimbursement Challenges: Limited insurance coverage for integrative services can pose challenges for individuals seeking these therapies. Advocacy for increased reimbursement for evidence-based integrative modalities is essential.

   - Affordability: The out-of-pocket costs associated with integrative therapies may be a barrier for some individuals, highlighting the need for increased accessibility and affordability.

3. Standardization of Practices:

   - Diverse Modalities: The diversity of integrative modalities makes standardization challenging. Establishing guidelines and best practices for various therapies is an ongoing effort within the field.

   - Education and Training: Ensuring that integrative healthcare providers receive comprehensive education and training in evidence-based practices is essential for maintaining quality care.

4. Cultural Competence:

   - Respecting Diverse Beliefs: Integrative medicine involves diverse cultural and belief systems. Practitioners must approach care with cultural competence, respecting individual beliefs and preferences.

   - Inclusion of Cultural Practices: Recognizing and incorporating cultural practices and traditions into integrative care plans enhances the relevance and effectiveness of these approaches.

Future Directions in Integrative Medicine Research

1. Effectiveness and Safety:

- Research on Modalities: Continued research on the safety and effectiveness of various integrative modalities is essential for building the evidence base and informing clinical practice.

- Longitudinal Studies: Longitudinal studies examining the impact of integrative approaches on chronic disease outcomes and long-term well-being contribute to the understanding of their efficacy.

2. Biomarker Development:

- Identification of Biomarkers: Exploring biomarkers associated with positive responses to integrative therapies allows for personalized treatment plans and enhances the precision of integrative care.

- Biosignatures of Well-Being: Identifying biosignatures associated with well-being and resilience provides insights into the physiological markers of positive health outcomes.

3. Digital Health Integration:

- Technology-Assisted Integrative Care: The integration of digital health tools, including mobile applications and telehealth platforms, expands access to integrative care and enhances patient engagement.

- Data Analytics: Analyzing data from digital health platforms contributes to the evaluation of treatment outcomes and the identification of patterns that inform personalized care.

4. Interdisciplinary Research Collaborations:

- Conventional and Integrative Partnerships: Collaborative research efforts involving conventional healthcare providers, integrative practitioners, and researchers contribute to the integration of evidence-based practices into mainstream care.

- Patient-Centered Outcomes Research: Incorporating patient perspectives and experiences into research design enhances the relevance and applicability of studies on integrative approaches.

Integrative approaches to treatment in chronic illness represent a transformative shift toward a more holistic and patient-centered paradigm. By recognizing the interconnectedness of physical, mental, and emotional well-being, integrative medicine aims to provide comprehensive care that addresses the diverse needs of individuals with chronic conditions. While challenges exist in terms of integration, standardization, and accessibility, ongoing research and collaborative efforts are shaping the future of integrative medicine. As the evidence base continues to expand and the integration of complementary therapies becomes more seamless within conventional care, individuals navigating chronic illnesses have the potential to experience a more comprehensive and personalized approach to their health and well-being.

Holistic Healing Modalities

Holistic healing modalities encompass a diverse array of practices that recognize the interconnected nature of the mind, body, and spirit in promoting overall well-being. Rooted in the belief that health is a dynamic balance within the individual and their environment, holistic approaches transcend conventional medical models by considering the totality of an individual's experience. From ancient practices to modern innovations, these modalities seek to address the underlying causes of imbalance, fostering not only the alleviation of symptoms but the cultivation of optimal health. This exploration delves into the principles, modalities, and potential benefits of holistic healing practices.

Principles of Holistic Healing

1. Wholeness and Integration:

   - Mind-Body-Spirit Connection: Holistic healing acknowledges the inseparable connection between the mind, body, and spirit. By addressing each of these aspects, practitioners aim to facilitate a state of wholeness and integration.

   - Unity of the Individual: Individuals are viewed as holistic entities, and health is seen as a reflection of the harmonious interplay of physical, mental, and spiritual dimensions.

2. Individualization and Personalization:

   - Unique Healing Journey: Holistic healing recognizes the individuality of each person's healing journey. Practices are tailored to the specific needs, preferences, and circumstances of the individual.

- Bioindividuality: Acknowledging that each person has unique biochemical and genetic makeups, holistic modalities take into account the diversity of responses to various interventions.

3. Prevention and Wellness Promotion:

- Proactive Health: Holistic healing emphasizes proactive approaches to health, placing a strong emphasis on prevention and wellness promotion.

- Lifestyle as Medicine: Lifestyle factors, including nutrition, exercise, stress management, and social connections, are considered foundational components of maintaining health and preventing illness.

4. Holistic Diagnosis and Treatment:

- Root Cause Analysis: Holistic healing seeks to identify and address the root causes of symptoms or imbalances rather than merely treating the symptoms.

- Comprehensive Assessment: Practitioners use a comprehensive assessment that considers physical, mental, emotional, and spiritual aspects to develop a holistic understanding of an individual's health.

Modalities of Holistic Healing

1. Traditional Chinese Medicine (TCM):

- Acupuncture: Acupuncture involves the insertion of thin needles into specific points on the body to balance the flow of energy, or Qi, and promote healing. It is used for a variety of conditions, including pain management, stress reduction, and fertility issues.

- Herbal Medicine: Chinese herbal medicine utilizes a variety of plant-based formulas to restore balance and address specific health concerns within the framework of TCM.

2. Ayurveda:

- Dosha Balancing: Ayurveda, an ancient system of medicine from India, identifies three doshas (Vata, Pitta, and Kapha) that govern individual constitution. Ayurvedic practices, including dietary adjustments, herbal remedies, and lifestyle recommendations, aim to balance these doshas for optimal health.

- Panchakarma: Panchakarma is a detoxification and rejuvenation process in Ayurveda, involving various therapeutic interventions to cleanse and revitalize the body.

3. Mind-Body Medicine:

- Mindfulness Meditation: Mindfulness meditation involves cultivating present-moment awareness and is used to reduce stress, improve mental focus, and enhance overall well-being.

- Biofeedback: Biofeedback is a technique that helps individuals gain awareness and control over physiological functions such as heart rate and muscle tension, promoting relaxation and stress reduction.

4. Energy Healing:

- Reiki: Reiki is a Japanese energy healing practice where practitioners channel universal life force energy to promote balance and facilitate the body's natural healing processes.

- Pranic Healing: Pranic healing involves the manipulation of energy (prana) to remove energetic blockages and restore health. It is based on the understanding that imbalances in the energy body precede physical ailments.

5. Holistic Nutrition:

- Functional Nutrition: Functional nutrition addresses the root causes of health issues by considering the interplay of diet, genetics, and lifestyle. It involves personalized dietary recommendations to support optimal health.

- Whole Foods and Plant-Based Diets: Emphasizing whole, nutrient-dense foods and plant-based diets is a holistic approach to nutrition that supports overall well-being and prevents illness.

6. Body-Mind Integration:

- Somatic Experiencing: Somatic experiencing focuses on the body's physical sensations to release and resolve the effects of trauma. It emphasizes the connection between the mind and the body in healing.

- Dance/Movement Therapy: Dance/movement therapy uses body movement and dance to promote emotional expression, self-awareness, and psychological well-being.

7. Herbalism:

- Western Herbalism: Western herbalism utilizes plants and botanicals to address a range of health issues. Herbalists may create custom herbal formulations based on an individual's specific needs.

- Adaptogens: Adaptogenic herbs, such as ginseng and ashwagandha, are used in herbal medicine to help the body adapt to stress and restore balance.

Benefits of Holistic Healing Modalities

1. Comprehensive Well-Being:

   - Mind-Body-Spirit Harmony: Holistic healing practices contribute to the harmony of the mind, body, and spirit, fostering a sense of overall well-being.

   - Improved Quality of Life: By addressing the root causes of imbalances, holistic modalities often lead to improvements in physical health, mental clarity, and emotional resilience.

2. Stress Reduction and Relaxation:

   - Cortisol Regulation: Practices such as meditation, biofeedback, and energy healing contribute to the regulation of cortisol levels, reducing the impact of chronic stress on the body.

   - Parasympathetic Activation: Holistic modalities activate the parasympathetic nervous system, promoting relaxation, rest, and recovery.

3. Chronic Pain Management:

   - Acupuncture: Acupuncture has been shown to be effective in managing chronic pain conditions, including back pain, osteoarthritis, and migraines.

   - Mind-Body Therapies: Mind-body practices, such as mindfulness and biofeedback, offer non-pharmacological approaches to chronic pain management.

4. Enhanced Mental Health:

   - Mindfulness-Based Approaches: Mindfulness meditation and other mindfulness-based practices have been associated with improvements in mental health, including reduced symptoms of anxiety and depression.

   - Therapeutic Movement Practices: Dance/movement therapy and somatic experiencing contribute to emotional expression and can be therapeutic for individuals dealing with mental health challenges.

5. Support for Chronic Conditions:

   - Autoimmune Disorders: Holistic approaches, including dietary modifications and stress reduction, may provide support for individuals with autoimmune conditions by addressing underlying inflammation.

   - Cardiovascular Health: Holistic nutrition and mind-body practices contribute to cardiovascular health by promoting healthy lifestyle habits and reducing risk factors.

6. Empowerment and Self-Care:

- Patient-Centered Care: Holistic healing modalities often involve a collaborative and empowering approach to care, encouraging individuals to actively participate in their healing journey.

- Mindful Self-Compassion: Mindfulness practices promote self-awareness and self-compassion, empowering individuals to cultivate a positive relationship with themselves.

Challenges and Considerations in Holistic Healing

1. Integration with Conventional Care:

- Communication and Collaboration: Integrating holistic healing modalities with conventional medical care requires effective communication and collaboration between practitioners from different fields.

- Evidence-Based Practices: Establishing evidence-based practices within the holistic healing community is essential for fostering trust and integration with mainstream healthcare.

2. Individual Variation in Response:

- Bioindividuality: Responses to holistic healing practices vary among individuals due to factors such as genetics, lifestyle, and personal beliefs.

- Trial and Error: Finding the most effective modalities for an individual may involve a process of trial and error, requiring patience and ongoing exploration.

3. Access and Affordability:

- Geographical Barriers: Access to certain holistic modalities may be limited by geographical location, especially in areas where these practices are not widely available.

- Costs of Services: Some holistic services may be out of reach for individuals with financial constraints, highlighting the need for increased accessibility and affordability.

4. Cultural Sensitivity:

- Cultural Perspectives: Holistic healing practices often draw from diverse cultural traditions. Practitioners must approach care with cultural sensitivity, respecting individual beliefs and practices.

- Inclusive Practices: Ensuring that holistic healing modalities are inclusive and respectful of cultural diversity contributes to their relevance and effectiveness.

Future Directions in Holistic Healing Research

1. Scientific Validation:

   - Research on Efficacy: Continued research on the efficacy of various holistic healing modalities is essential for building the evidence base and establishing these practices within the realm of evidence-based medicine.

   - Mechanisms of Action: Understanding the mechanisms of action behind holistic modalities contributes to the scientific validation of their effectiveness.

2. Integrative Models of Care:

   - Interdisciplinary Research: Collaborative research efforts involving practitioners from diverse fields, including conventional and holistic medicine, contribute to the development of integrative models of care.

   - Patient-Centered Outcomes Research: Incorporating patient perspectives and experiences into research design enhances the relevance and applicability of studies on holistic healing.

3. Digital Health Integration:

   - Telehealth for Holistic Care: The integration of holistic healing practices into telehealth platforms expands access to these modalities, allowing individuals to receive care remotely.

   - Digital Platforms for Education: Digital platforms offer opportunities for education and awareness about holistic healing, promoting informed decision-making among individuals seeking these modalities.

4. Community-Based Approaches:

   - Public Health Initiatives: Community-based initiatives that promote holistic approaches to health, including education and accessible services, contribute to improved public health outcomes.

   - Collaboration with Communities: Collaborative efforts involving healthcare professionals, community leaders, and individuals enhance the effectiveness of community-based approaches.

Embracing Holistic Well-Being

Holistic healing modalities provide a rich tapestry of approaches that honor the complexity of human experience and well-being. From ancient traditions to contemporary innovations, these practices contribute to the cultivation of holistic health by addressing the interconnected dimensions of mind, body, and spirit. As research advances and integrative models of care become more prevalent, individuals navigating their healing journeys have the opportunity to embrace a holistic approach that recognizes the inherent wisdom of the body and the potential for transformative well-being. By fostering collaboration, inclusivity, and ongoing research, the landscape of holistic healing continues to evolve, offering a diverse array of tools to support individuals on their paths to optimal health and vitality.

CHAPTER EIGHT

Lifestyle Modifications for Disease Prevention

The global burden of chronic diseases continues to rise, and many of these conditions are closely linked to lifestyle factors. While genetics play a role in disease susceptibility, lifestyle modifications have emerged as a powerful tool for preventing and managing various health conditions. This comprehensive exploration delves into the intricate interplay between lifestyle choices and disease prevention, examining the impact of diet, physical activity, sleep, stress management, and other factors on overall health and well-being.

Diet: Nourishing the Body, Defending Against Disease

Diet is a cornerstone of health, influencing the risk of developing numerous chronic conditions. Adopting a balanced and nutrient-rich diet can significantly contribute to disease prevention.

1. Mediterranean Diet: The Mediterranean diet, characterized by a high intake of fruits, vegetables, whole grains, and olive oil, has been extensively studied for its health benefits.

   - Cardiovascular Health:Rich in monounsaturated fats, the Mediterranean diet has been associated with a reduced risk of cardiovascular diseases.

   - Cancer Prevention:Antioxidant-rich foods in this diet, such as fruits and vegetables, may contribute to a lower risk of certain cancers.

2. Plant-Based Diets: Plant-based diets, whether vegetarian or vegan, emphasize plant-derived foods while minimizing or excluding animal products.

   - Heart Health: Plant-based diets are linked to lower blood pressure, cholesterol levels, and a reduced risk of heart disease.

   - Type 2 Diabetes Prevention: A plant-based diet may contribute to better blood sugar control, reducing the risk of type 2 diabetes.

3. Anti-Inflammatory Eating: Chronic inflammation is implicated in various diseases, and certain foods can either promote or mitigate inflammation.

   - Omega-3 Fatty Acids: Found in fatty fish, flaxseeds, and walnuts, omega-3 fatty acids have anti-inflammatory properties.

   - Turmeric and Ginger: These spices contain compounds with anti-inflammatory effects and are used in traditional medicine for their health benefits.

4. Mindful Eating: Beyond the content of the diet, how and when one eats can impact health.

- Portion Control: Overeating contributes to obesity, a risk factor for numerous diseases.

- Eating Patterns: Intermittent fasting and time-restricted eating patterns are being investigated for their potential health benefits, including metabolic improvements and longevity.

Physical Activity: A Pillar of Disease Prevention

Regular physical activity is a cornerstone of a healthy lifestyle, offering protection against a myriad of chronic conditions.

1. Cardiovascular Exercise: Aerobic activities such as walking, running, cycling, and swimming benefit the cardiovascular system.

- Heart Health: Regular cardiovascular exercise improves heart health, reducing the risk of heart disease and stroke.

- Blood Pressure Management: Exercise contributes to lower blood pressure, a crucial factor in preventing hypertension.

2. Strength Training: Building and maintaining muscle mass through strength training exercises provide various health benefits.

- Bone Health: Resistance training helps maintain bone density, reducing the risk of osteoporosis.

- Metabolic Health: Increased muscle mass contributes to better metabolic health, aiding in weight management and glucose control.

3. Flexibility and Balance Exercises: Activities that enhance flexibility and balance, such as yoga and tai chi, are valuable for overall well-being.

- Fall Prevention: Improving balance reduces the risk of falls, particularly in older adults.

- Stress Reduction: Mind-body exercises like yoga promote relaxation and stress management.

Sleep Hygiene: Unveiling the Healing Powers of Rest

Adequate and quality sleep is integral to physical and mental health, playing a crucial role in disease prevention.

1. Sleep Duration: The recommended amount of sleep varies across age groups, but consistently obtaining sufficient sleep is associated with numerous health benefits.

- Cognitive Function: Sleep is vital for cognitive processes such as memory consolidation and learning.

- Immune Function: Adequate sleep supports a robust immune system, reducing susceptibility to infections.

2. Sleep Quality: Beyond duration, the quality of sleep is paramount for its health-promoting effects.

- Mood Regulation: Quality sleep contributes to emotional well-being and helps regulate mood.

- Chronic Disease Risk: Poor sleep is associated with an increased risk of conditions like obesity, diabetes, and cardiovascular diseases.

Stress Management: Balancing the Scales of Well-being

Chronic stress is implicated in the pathogenesis of various diseases, making stress management a crucial aspect of disease prevention.

1. Mindfulness Meditation: Mindfulness practices, including meditation and deep-breathing exercises, promote relaxation and stress reduction.

- Cortisol Regulation: Mindfulness meditation has been associated with lower levels of cortisol, a stress hormone.

- Anxiety and Depression: Mindfulness-based interventions show promise in alleviating symptoms of anxiety and depression.

2. Yoga and Tai Chi: Mind-body exercises like yoga and tai chi combine physical activity with meditative elements, offering holistic benefits.

- Muscle Relaxation: These practices promote physical relaxation, reducing tension and muscle stiffness.

- Improved Sleep: Regular practice is linked to better sleep quality, further contributing to overall well-being.

3. Social Connections: Social support and strong interpersonal relationships play a pivotal role in stress management.

- Emotional Support: Having a robust social network provides emotional support during challenging times.

- Health Behaviors: Social connections influence health behaviors, encouraging positive lifestyle choices.

Tobacco and Alcohol: Breaking Free from Detrimental Habits

Tobacco and excessive alcohol consumption are major contributors to various diseases, and cessation or moderation is key to disease prevention.

1. Smoking Cessation: Quitting smoking is one of the most impactful lifestyle changes for preventing a myriad of diseases.

   - Cardiovascular Health: The risk of heart disease and stroke decreases significantly after smoking cessation.

   - Cancer Prevention: The link between smoking and various cancers underscores the importance of quitting.

2. Moderate Alcohol Consumption: While moderate alcohol consumption may have some health benefits, excessive intake poses significant risks.

   - Heart Health: Moderate alcohol consumption is associated with a reduced risk of heart disease.

   - Liver Health: Excessive alcohol consumption can lead to liver diseases, emphasizing the importance of moderation.

Screen Time and Mental Health: Striking a Balance in the Digital Age

Excessive screen time, particularly on electronic devices, has become ubiquitous in the modern era and is linked to various health concerns.

1. Digital Detox: Limiting screen time and taking breaks from electronic devices is crucial for mental and physical well-being.

   - Eye Health: Prolonged screen time can lead to digital eye strain and other visual discomforts.

   - Sleep Quality: Blue light emitted by screens can disrupt sleep patterns, underscoring the importance of minimizing screen exposure before bedtime.

2. Social Media and Mental Health: The impact of social media on mental health is a growing area of concern.

   - Comparison and Self-Esteem: Constant exposure to curated content can contribute to social comparison and impact self-esteem.

   - Positive Connections: While there are potential negatives, social media can also facilitate positive connections and support networks.

Regular Health Check-ups: Proactive Monitoring for Early Intervention

Regular health check-ups and screenings are instrumental in early detection and prevention of diseases.

1. Preventive Screenings: Screening tests for conditions such as cancer, diabetes, and hypertension enable early intervention.

   - Cancer Screening: Mammograms, colonoscopies, and Pap smears are examples of screenings that can detect cancer in its early stages.

   - Blood Pressure and Cholesterol Checks: Monitoring blood pressure and cholesterol levels aids in preventing cardiovascular diseases.

2. Vaccinations: Vaccinations are a critical component of disease prevention, protecting against infectious diseases.

   - Childhood Vaccines: Routine childhood vaccinations prevent diseases such as measles, mumps, and polio.

   - Adult Vaccines: Influenza, pneumonia, and shingles vaccines are examples of immunizations recommended for adults.

Environmental Factors: Nurturing a Health-Promoting Environment

Environmental factors, both external and internal, play a role in overall health, and making conscious choices in this regard contributes to disease prevention.

1. Clean Air and Water: Access to clean air and water is fundamental for health, and efforts to minimize exposure to pollutants are crucial.

   - Respiratory Health: Air pollution can contribute to respiratory diseases, making efforts to reduce exposure vital.

   - Water Quality: Access to safe drinking water is essential for preventing waterborne diseases.

2. Occupational Health: Occupational exposures can impact health, and measures to promote workplace safety are essential.

   - Ergonomics: Proper ergonomic practices contribute to musculoskeletal health and prevent workplace injuries.

- Chemical Exposures: Awareness and control of chemical exposures in the workplace are critical for preventing occupational diseases.

Community Engagement: Fostering Health at a Societal Level

Engaging with the community and advocating for health-promoting policies contribute to disease prevention on a broader scale.

1. Community Health Programs: Community-based initiatives can address health disparities and promote overall well-being.

   - Health Education: Community health programs can provide education on nutrition, exercise, and disease prevention.

   - Access to Healthcare: Initiatives that enhance healthcare access contribute to preventive care and early intervention.

2. Advocacy for Health Policies: Advocacy for policies that promote public health is a powerful tool for disease prevention.

   - Tobacco Control: Policies such as tobacco taxes and smoking bans contribute to reduced tobacco use.

   - Healthy Food Initiatives: Supporting policies that promote access to healthy foods helps combat obesity and diet-related diseases.

A Lifelong Commitment to Health

Lifestyle modifications for disease prevention encompass a diverse array of choices, each playing a unique role in shaping overall health and well-being. From dietary patterns to physical activity, sleep hygiene, and stress management, every aspect of lifestyle contributes to the intricate tapestry of disease prevention.

Adopting a holistic approach that considers individual needs, preferences, and cultural factors is paramount. Moreover, disease prevention is a lifelong commitment, requiring ongoing awareness, education, and adaptation to changing circumstances. As we navigate the complexities of modern life, the power to prevent disease lies within the choices we make every day, empowering individuals to take charge of their health and cultivate a life rich in vitality and well-being.

Public Health Initiatives

Public health initiatives represent a collective and systematic effort to improve the health and well-being of entire populations. Rooted in the principles of prevention, equity, and community engagement, these initiatives address a spectrum of health determinants, from infectious diseases and chronic conditions to environmental factors and social disparities. This exploration delves into the multifaceted realm of public health initiatives, examining their objectives, strategies, and the impact they have on fostering healthier communities.

Understanding Public Health Initiatives

1. Defining Public Health: A Holistic Perspective

Public health goes beyond individual medical care to focus on the health of entire populations. It encompasses a wide range of activities and interventions designed to prevent disease, promote health, and address the underlying factors that influence well-being.

Prevention is a central theme in public health, encompassing primary prevention (preventing diseases before they occur), secondary prevention (early detection and intervention), and tertiary prevention (minimizing the impact of existing conditions).

Public health initiatives recognize that health outcomes are influenced by social, economic, and environmental factors. Addressing these determinants is essential for creating equitable health opportunities.

2. The Objectives of Public Health Initiatives

Public health initiatives are guided by a set of overarching objectives aimed at improving health outcomes and creating conditions that support well-being across diverse populations.

Targeting infectious diseases, chronic conditions, and emerging health threats through vaccination campaigns, health screenings, and education initiatives.

Encouraging healthy behaviors, such as physical activity, proper nutrition, and tobacco cessation, to enhance overall well-being and prevent lifestyle-related diseases.

Promoting fairness and eliminating health disparities by addressing social determinants of health and ensuring that all individuals have equal access to healthcare resources and opportunities.

Safeguarding communities from environmental hazards, ensuring access to clean air and water, and promoting sustainable practices to protect the planet and public health.Building resilience and response capabilities to address public health emergencies, including natural disasters, pandemics, and other crises.

Strategies in Public Health Initiatives

1. Health Education and Communication: Empowering Communities

Effective communication is fundamental to public health initiatives, empowering individuals and communities with knowledge and resources to make informed health decisions.

Designing and implementing initiatives that enhance health literacy, ensuring that individuals can understand and act upon health information to make informed choices.

Utilizing various media channels to disseminate health messages, promote preventive behaviors, and raise awareness about specific health issues, from vaccination campaigns to anti-smoking initiatives.

Engaging with diverse communities through targeted outreach programs, culturally sensitive materials, and community partnerships to ensure that health messages resonate with different populations.

2. Vaccination Campaigns: Preventing Infectious Diseases

Vaccination is a cornerstone of public health, preventing the spread of infectious diseases and protecting communities from outbreaks.

Implementing and promoting routine vaccination schedules to ensure that individuals receive timely and appropriate vaccines throughout their lifespan.

Rapid deployment of vaccination campaigns during outbreaks of vaccine-preventable diseases to control the spread and protect vulnerable populations.

Communicating the importance of vaccination to the public, dispelling myths, and addressing concerns to foster widespread acceptance and participation.

3. Healthcare Access and Equity: Ensuring Inclusive Services

Public health initiatives aim to enhance access to quality healthcare services, with a focus on reaching underserved and marginalized populations.

Establishing and supporting community health clinics that provide essential services, including preventive care, screenings, and education, particularly in areas with limited access to healthcare facilities.

Deploying mobile health units to bring healthcare services directly to communities, addressing geographical barriers and reaching populations with limited transportation options.

Expanding telehealth services to increase access to medical consultations, particularly in rural or remote areas, and improving healthcare delivery efficiency.

4. Community-Based Interventions: Tailoring Approaches to Local Needs

Public health initiatives are most effective when they are designed with the specific needs and contexts of communities in mind.

Conducting thorough assessments to identify the unique health challenges, resources, and cultural factors within a community, informing the development of targeted interventions.

Implementing programs that empower communities to take an active role in their health, fostering a sense of ownership and sustainability.

Designing interventions that respect and incorporate the cultural diversity of communities, ensuring that strategies are inclusive and resonate with different cultural backgrounds.

5. Policy Advocacy: Shaping Environments for Health

Public health initiatives often involve advocating for policy changes that create environments supportive of health and well-being.

Implementing and advocating for policies such as smoking bans, tobacco taxation, and graphic warning labels to reduce tobacco use and its associated health risks.

Supporting policies that promote access to healthy foods, regulate food labeling, and address issues such as food deserts to improve nutrition and prevent obesity.

Advocating for and enforcing regulations that protect air and water quality, control exposure to hazardous substances, and promote sustainable practices for a healthier environment.

Impact and Challenges in Public Health Initiatives

1. Measuring Impact: Assessing Health Outcomes

Evaluating the success of public health initiatives involves monitoring key health indicators, measuring the prevalence of diseases, and assessing changes in health behaviors within populations.

Implementing robust surveillance systems to track disease prevalence, monitor health trends, and identify emerging health threats for timely intervention.

Evaluating the impact of interventions by assessing changes in health outcomes, such as reductions in disease incidence, improvements in vaccination rates, and positive shifts in health behaviors.

Recognizing that the impact of public health initiatives may manifest over the long term, necessitating sustained efforts and continuous monitoring to gauge success.

2. Global Collaboration: Addressing Transnational Health Challenges

Many health challenges transcend borders, necessitating global collaboration and coordination to effectively address issues such as infectious disease outbreaks and the impact of climate change on health.

Collaborating with organizations such as the World Health Organization (WHO) to share information, coordinate responses to global health threats, and promote best practices in public health.

Facilitating international research collaborations and sharing data to enhance understanding of global health trends, identify common challenges, and develop effective strategies.

Providing assistance during public health emergencies, natural disasters, and conflicts to ensure that affected populations receive necessary healthcare services and support.

3. Challenges and Considerations: Navigating Complexities

Despite the positive impact of public health initiatives, various challenges and considerations must be navigated to optimize effectiveness and inclusivity.

Balancing limited resources with the diverse health needs of populations, requiring strategic prioritization and efficient use of available funding.

Garnering political support and advocacy to ensure the implementation of evidence-based public health policies and interventions.

Fostering genuine community engagement to ensure that interventions are culturally sensitive, well-received, and reflective of the needs and preferences of diverse populations.

Developing targeted interventions to address health disparities and inequities, recognizing that different populations may face unique challenges in accessing healthcare and achieving optimal health outcomes.

Future Directions in Public Health Initiatives

1. Advancements in Technology: Harnessing Digital Solutions

Technology offers new avenues for enhancing the reach and impact of public health initiatives, from data analytics and telehealth to mobile applications and digital communication platforms.

Leveraging data analytics and artificial intelligence for real-time surveillance, early detection of health trends, and timely intervention during outbreaks.

Expanding telehealth services to increase access to healthcare, particularly in underserved areas, and improving the efficiency of healthcare delivery.

Developing and promoting mobile applications that provide health information, support behavior change, and facilitate remote monitoring for chronic conditions.

2. Climate Change and Health: Integrating Environmental Considerations

The intersection of climate change and public health is an emerging area of focus, requiring a holistic approach to address the health impacts of environmental shifts.

Developing and implementing public health strategies to adapt to the health impacts of climate change, such as changes in disease patterns, extreme weather events, and food security.

Promoting environmentally sustainable practices in healthcare, urban planning, and agriculture to mitigate the impact of human activities on climate and health.

Raising awareness about the health implications of climate change and advocating for policies that prioritize both environmental sustainability and public health.

3. Pandemic Preparedness: Strengthening Global Resilience

The COVID-19 pandemic underscored the importance of global preparedness for pandemics and other health emergencies, prompting a renewed focus on building resilience.

Promoting equitable access to vaccines worldwide to ensure widespread immunity and prevent the emergence and spread of infectious diseases.

Strengthening international collaboration in surveillance, data sharing, and response coordination to address pandemics collectively.

Investing in research and innovation to develop new tools, technologies, and strategies for pandemic prevention, preparedness, and response.

Building Healthier Communities Together

Public health initiatives represent a shared commitment to creating conditions that allow individuals and communities to thrive. By addressing the root causes of health disparities, promoting preventive measures, and fostering inclusive and equitable approaches, public health initiatives contribute to the building of healthier communities. The challenges and complexities inherent in public health require ongoing collaboration, innovation, and a commitment to addressing the evolving health needs of diverse populations. As we navigate the path toward a healthier future, the collective efforts of policymakers, healthcare professionals, communities, and individuals are essential to ensuring that public health initiatives continue to make a meaningful and lasting impact on the well-being of societies worldwide.

CHAPTER NINE

Strengthening the Body's Natural Defenses

The human body is equipped with a remarkable defense system that safeguards it against a myriad of pathogens, toxins, and environmental threats. This intricate network of defenses includes physical barriers, immune cells, and various physiological processes working in harmony to maintain health and well-being. Strengthening the body's natural defenses is crucial for maintaining optimal health and preventing illnesses. In this comprehensive exploration, we delve into the multifaceted ways through which individuals can enhance and support their innate defense mechanisms.

A balanced and nutrient-rich diet is the cornerstone of a robust immune system. Essential vitamins and minerals play a pivotal role in supporting various immune functions. Vitamin C, found in citrus fruits and leafy greens, is known for its antioxidant properties and its role in enhancing immune cell function. Vitamin D, obtained from sunlight exposure and certain foods, is crucial for immune regulation. Incorporating a diverse range of fruits, vegetables, whole grains, and lean proteins provides the body with the necessary nutrients to bolster its defenses.

Proper hydration is often underestimated in its role in immune health. Water is essential for various bodily functions, including the transport of nutrients, elimination of waste products, and the maintenance of optimal body temperature. Staying adequately hydrated ensures that these processes operate smoothly, supporting the body's overall well-being and immune function.

Regular physical activity has been consistently linked to improved immune function. Exercise promotes the circulation of immune cells, helping them to reach different parts of the body efficiently. It also contributes to the reduction of chronic inflammation, a factor associated with various diseases. Engaging in a mix of cardiovascular exercises, strength training, and flexibility exercises can contribute to a well-rounded approach to fitness and immune support.

Adequate and quality sleep is fundamental for the body's recovery and immune function. During sleep, the body undergoes various processes that repair tissues and consolidate memories. Sleep deprivation has been shown to impair immune responses, making individuals more susceptible to infections. Establishing a regular sleep routine and creating a conducive sleep environment are essential steps in fortifying the body's natural defenses.

Chronic stress can have detrimental effects on the immune system. Stress hormones, such as cortisol, can suppress immune function over time. Incorporating stress-reduction techniques, such

as meditation, deep breathing exercises, or yoga, into daily life can help manage stress levels and promote a healthier immune response.

Basic hygiene practices are critical for preventing the spread of infections and supporting the body's natural defenses. Regular handwashing, proper food handling, and maintaining cleanliness in living spaces help reduce the risk of exposure to harmful pathogens. These practices form the first line of defense against infections.

The gut plays a pivotal role in immune function, housing a significant portion of the body's immune cells. Probiotics, beneficial bacteria found in fermented foods and supplements, contribute to a healthy gut microbiome. A balanced and diverse microbiome supports immune function and helps prevent the overgrowth of harmful bacteria. Including probiotic-rich foods, such as yogurt and kefir, in the diet can positively impact gut health.

Certain herbs and adaptogens have been traditionally used to support immune health. Echinacea, elderberry, and astragalus are examples of herbs with immune-boosting properties. Adaptogens like ashwagandha and rhodiola help the body adapt to stress, potentially reducing the negative impact of chronic stress on the immune system. While these supplements can be beneficial, it's essential to consult with a healthcare professional before incorporating them into one's routine.

Vaccination is a crucial aspect of strengthening the body's defenses against specific pathogens. Vaccines train the immune system to recognize and combat harmful microorganisms, providing protection against infectious diseases. Staying up-to-date with recommended vaccinations is an effective strategy for preventing certain illnesses and maintaining overall health.

Social connections and a strong support network contribute to mental and emotional well-being, which, in turn, positively influences immune function. Maintaining meaningful relationships, participating in social activities, and having a support system during challenging times can help reduce stress and promote a healthier immune response.

In conclusion, strengthening the body's natural defenses involves adopting a holistic approach that addresses various aspects of lifestyle and well-being. A nutrient-rich diet, regular exercise, adequate sleep, stress management, and proper hygiene practices form the foundation of a robust immune system. Supplementing these lifestyle measures with vaccinations, probiotics, and herbal supplements can further enhance immune health. By incorporating these practices into daily life, individuals can empower their bodies to better defend against the constant challenges posed by the environment and potential pathogens. Ultimately, a proactive and comprehensive approach to immune support is key to maintaining optimal health and well-being throughout life.

Cultivating Mental and Emotional Well-being

In the fast-paced and demanding world we live in, cultivating mental and emotional well-being has become increasingly vital. The intricate interplay between the mind and emotions significantly influences our overall health and quality of life. This comprehensive exploration delves into the multifaceted aspects of mental and emotional well-being, examining the factors that contribute to it and offering practical strategies for fostering resilience, self-awareness, and emotional balance.

Mental and emotional well-being encompass a broad spectrum of factors that contribute to an individual's psychological health. Mental well-being involves cognitive functions, such as clarity of thought, effective problem-solving, and the ability to cope with stress. Emotional well-being, on the other hand, pertains to the awareness and regulation of emotions, as well as the capacity to form and maintain positive relationships.

Self-awareness is a foundational element of mental and emotional well-being. It involves recognizing and understanding one's thoughts, feelings, and behaviors. Cultivating self-awareness provides individuals with insights into their motivations, strengths, and areas for growth. Practices such as mindfulness meditation, journaling, and regular self-reflection can enhance self-awareness, fostering a deeper connection with one's inner self.

Emotional regulation is the ability to manage and modulate one's emotional responses. It involves recognizing emotions as they arise and responding to them in a healthy and constructive manner. Techniques like deep breathing, progressive muscle relaxation, and cognitive-behavioral strategies can help individuals regulate their emotions, preventing the negative impact of overwhelming feelings on mental well-being.

Resilience is the capacity to bounce back from adversity and navigate challenges with a positive outlook. Building resilience involves developing coping mechanisms, fostering a growth mindset, and cultivating a sense of optimism. Learning from setbacks, maintaining a sense of perspective, and seeking support when needed contribute to the development of resilience, which is a crucial aspect of long-term mental well-being.

Healthy and positive relationships are integral to emotional well-being. Social connections provide emotional support, companionship, and a sense of belonging. Nurturing meaningful relationships with family, friends, and community members can positively impact mental health. Effective communication, empathy, and the ability to set boundaries contribute to the creation and maintenance of positive connections.

Stress is an inevitable part of life, but effective stress management is key to maintaining mental and emotional well-being. Adopting stress-reduction techniques such as regular exercise, mindfulness practices, and time management can mitigate the negative effects of chronic stress. Balancing work and personal life, setting realistic goals, and learning to delegate tasks are practical strategies for reducing stressors.

Physical and mental well-being are interconnected, and lifestyle choices play a significant role in both. Regular physical activity has been shown to have positive effects on mood and cognitive function. Adequate sleep is crucial for cognitive functioning, emotional regulation, and overall mental health. Additionally, a balanced diet rich in nutrients supports brain function and provides the energy needed for daily activities.

Engaging in lifelong learning and pursuing personal growth contribute to a sense of purpose and fulfillment. Whether through formal education, skill development, or pursuing hobbies, continuous learning fosters cognitive stimulation and creativity. Setting and achieving personal goals provide a sense of accomplishment, boosting self-esteem and contributing to overall mental well-being.

Mindfulness practices, including meditation, have gained recognition for their positive impact on mental and emotional well-being. Mindfulness involves paying attention to the present moment without judgment. Regular meditation practice has been associated with reduced stress, improved focus, and increased emotional resilience. Mindfulness-based interventions, such as Mindfulness-Based Stress Reduction (MBSR), are widely used to enhance well-being.

Acknowledging the importance of seeking professional support is a sign of strength, not weakness. Mental health professionals, including psychologists, counselors, and psychiatrists, are trained to provide support and guidance. Therapy can help individuals explore and address underlying issues, develop coping strategies, and gain valuable insights into their thoughts and emotions.

Cultivating a sense of gratitude involves consciously acknowledging and appreciating the positive aspects of life. Gratitude practices, such as keeping a gratitude journal or expressing appreciation to others, have been linked to increased feelings of well-being. Focusing on what one is grateful for can shift the perspective from what is lacking to what is present, promoting a positive outlook.

In conclusion, cultivating mental and emotional well-being is a multifaceted journey that encompasses various aspects of life. It involves self-awareness, emotional regulation, resilience, positive relationships, stress management, healthy lifestyle choices, lifelong learning, mindfulness, seeking professional support, and gratitude practices. By incorporating these elements into daily life, individuals can create a foundation for lasting mental and emotional well-being.

It's important to recognize that mental health is a dynamic and evolving aspect of human experience. What works for one person may not work for another, and the journey to well-being is unique for each individual. As society continues to evolve, so too does our understanding of mental health, emphasizing the need for ongoing dialogue, compassion, and support for those navigating the complexities of the mind and emotions. Ultimately, prioritizing mental and emotional well-being is an investment in the overall quality of life, fostering resilience, fulfillment, and a sense of purpose.

CHAPTER TEN

Innovations in Medicine and Wellness

The field of medicine and wellness is experiencing a transformative era marked by groundbreaking innovations that have the potential to revolutionize healthcare. From advancements in medical technologies to novel approaches in preventive care, these innovations are reshaping how we approach health and well-being. This comprehensive exploration delves into the latest innovations in medicine and wellness, examining their impact on patient care, disease prevention, and the overall landscape of healthcare.

Precision medicine, also known as personalized medicine, is a revolutionary approach to medical treatment and healthcare that takes into account individual differences in patients' genes, environments, and lifestyles. It involves tailoring medical care and treatments to the specific characteristics of each patient, allowing for more precise and effective interventions. Advances in genomics, molecular biology, and data analytics have paved the way for a deeper understanding of the genetic basis of diseases, enabling healthcare providers to develop targeted therapies and interventions.

Telemedicine has emerged as a transformative force in healthcare, particularly in the context of providing remote access to medical services. Telemedicine allows patients to consult with healthcare professionals through virtual platforms, breaking down geographical barriers and improving accessibility to care. Additionally, remote patient monitoring technologies enable continuous tracking of vital signs and health metrics, allowing for early detection of health issues and timely interventions. This shift towards virtual healthcare has proven especially crucial during global health crises, enhancing the efficiency and accessibility of medical services.

Artificial intelligence (AI) is making significant inroads into the field of medicine, offering innovative solutions for diagnosis, treatment planning, and patient care. Machine learning algorithms analyze vast datasets, including medical images, patient records, and clinical studies, to identify patterns and correlations that may not be apparent to human practitioners. AI applications range from early detection of diseases through image recognition to personalized treatment recommendations based on individual patient data. As AI continues to evolve, its integration into healthcare systems holds the promise of improving diagnostic accuracy, treatment outcomes, and overall efficiency.

The application of 3D printing technology in healthcare is expanding rapidly, offering new possibilities for personalized medical devices, prosthetics, and even organs. 3D printing allows for the creation of intricate and customized structures based on patient-specific data. In orthopedics, for example, 3D printing is used to produce implants tailored to the unique anatomy of individual patients. Researchers are also exploring the potential of bioprinting, a specialized form of 3D

printing, to generate functional tissues and organs for transplantation, addressing the critical issue of organ shortages.

Immunotherapy represents a paradigm shift in the treatment of cancer and other diseases by harnessing the body's own immune system to combat illness. This innovative approach involves stimulating or modulating the immune response to target and destroy abnormal cells. In cancer treatment, immunotherapies such as checkpoint inhibitors and CAR-T cell therapy have shown remarkable success in certain cases, providing new hope for patients with previously untreatable conditions. Ongoing research in immunotherapy is exploring its potential applications in various autoimmune disorders and infectious diseases.

Nanomedicine involves the use of nanotechnology for medical applications, offering precise and targeted interventions at the molecular and cellular levels. Nanoparticles, ranging in size from 1 to 100 nanometers, can be engineered to deliver drugs directly to specific cells or tissues, minimizing side effects and enhancing therapeutic efficacy. In diagnostics, nanoscale sensors and imaging agents enable early detection of diseases. The field of nanomedicine holds promise for revolutionizing drug delivery, imaging, and diagnostics, opening new avenues for more effective and personalized medical interventions.

Advancements in robotic technology have led to the development of robotic-assisted surgery, a minimally invasive approach that allows surgeons to perform complex procedures with enhanced precision and control. Robotic surgical systems, such as the da Vinci Surgical System, enable surgeons to manipulate robotic arms with greater dexterity and accuracy, leading to smaller incisions, reduced recovery times, and improved patient outcomes. The integration of augmented reality and virtual reality technologies further enhances surgical planning and training, pushing the boundaries of what is possible in modern surgical practice.

Blockchain technology, known for its secure and transparent decentralized ledger system, is finding applications in healthcare for data management and security. The use of blockchain can streamline the sharing and access of patient records, ensuring data integrity and interoperability across different healthcare providers. Patients can have greater control over their health data, granting permission for specific parties to access their information. Blockchain also holds promise in areas such as drug traceability, clinical trials, and the prevention of counterfeit medications.

The proliferation of smartphones has given rise to a plethora of health and wellness apps designed to empower individuals in managing their well-being. These apps cover a wide range of functions, from fitness tracking and nutrition monitoring to mental health support and medication management. Mobile health (mHealth) applications have the potential to promote preventive care, encourage healthy lifestyles, and provide valuable data for both patients and healthcare providers. Integrating these apps into patient care plans can contribute to more proactive and patient-centered approaches to wellness.

Gene editing technologies, such as CRISPR-Cas9, have revolutionized the field of genetics by allowing precise modification of DNA sequences. While still in the early stages of application, gene editing holds promise for treating genetic disorders by correcting or modifying faulty genes. The potential to edit genes associated with conditions like cystic fibrosis and sickle cell anemia

has generated considerable excitement in the scientific and medical communities. Ethical considerations and ongoing research into the safety and efficacy of gene editing technologies remain central to their future implementation.

In conclusion, the landscape of medicine and wellness is undergoing a profound transformation fueled by innovative technologies and approaches. Precision medicine, telemedicine, artificial intelligence, 3D printing, immunotherapy, nanomedicine, robotic surgery, blockchain, health apps, and gene editing are among the cutting-edge developments shaping the future of healthcare. These innovations hold the promise of more personalized, efficient, and accessible medical care, with the potential to revolutionize how we approach health and well-being on both individual and societal levels.

As these technologies continue to evolve, it is essential for healthcare professionals, policymakers, and the public to collaborate in navigating the ethical, regulatory, and societal implications of these innovations. Striking a balance between embracing the benefits of medical and wellness advancements and addressing potential challenges is crucial for ensuring that these innovations contribute positively to the well-being of individuals and communities. The ongoing pursuit of knowledge, ethical considerations, and a commitment to accessibility and inclusivity will be key in harnessing the full potential of these innovations for the betterment of global health.

A Roadmap for a Healthier Society

Building a healthier society is a multifaceted and complex endeavor that requires a comprehensive roadmap addressing various aspects of individual and collective well-being. The quest for a healthier society involves not only the absence of illness but also the promotion of physical, mental, and social well-being. In this exploration, we embark on a journey to outline a roadmap for creating and sustaining a healthier society, encompassing healthcare, education, community engagement, and policy interventions.

A cornerstone of a healthier society is a healthcare system that is not only accessible to all but also prioritizes equity. Accessible healthcare involves removing barriers that prevent individuals from seeking and receiving medical attention. This includes addressing geographical disparities, ensuring affordability, and eliminating discriminatory practices. Equity, on the other hand, emphasizes fair and just distribution of resources and opportunities. A healthier society recognizes the importance of preventive care, early intervention, and ongoing support for all its members, irrespective of socioeconomic status, race, or other factors.

Preventive healthcare plays a pivotal role in reducing the burden of illness and promoting overall well-being. Public health initiatives focused on preventive measures, such as vaccinations, health screenings, and lifestyle education, contribute to a healthier population. By emphasizing the importance of healthy behaviors, early detection of risk factors, and community-wide interventions, societies can reduce the prevalence of preventable diseases and create a culture of proactive health management.

A healthier society recognizes the significance of mental health and places it on par with physical health. Mental health support should be integrated into healthcare systems, workplaces, and educational institutions. This includes destigmatizing mental health issues, providing accessible and affordable mental health services, and fostering a supportive community environment. Education and awareness campaigns can play a crucial role in promoting mental health literacy, helping individuals recognize, understand, and address mental health concerns effectively.

Education is a powerful tool for building a healthier society. A holistic approach to education goes beyond traditional academic subjects and includes health literacy as a core component. Health education should cover topics such as nutrition, physical activity, mental health, and preventive care. Integrating these subjects into curricula from an early age helps equip individuals with the knowledge and skills needed to make informed decisions about their health. Furthermore, education should promote critical thinking, resilience, and social-emotional learning to support overall well-being.

A sense of community and social support is fundamental to individual and collective well-being. A healthier society encourages active community engagement, fostering social connections, and creating networks of support. Community-based initiatives, such as wellness programs, local events, and support groups, can strengthen social ties and provide individuals with a sense of belonging. By nurturing inclusive and supportive communities, societies can address social determinants of health and promote a sense of shared responsibility for well-being.

The physical environment in which people live, work, and play significantly influences their health. Healthy urban planning and infrastructure design prioritize walkability, green spaces, and accessibility to healthcare facilities. Creating environments that facilitate physical activity, reduce air pollution, and promote sustainable living contributes to a healthier society. Urban planning should also consider factors such as affordable housing, safe neighborhoods, and public transportation to address social determinants of health and create equitable opportunities for all residents.

The workplace is a crucial setting for promoting health and well-being, considering the amount of time individuals spend on the job. Employers play a key role in creating a healthy work environment by implementing workplace wellness programs. These programs can include fitness initiatives, mental health resources, ergonomic support, and incentives for healthy behaviors. By prioritizing employee well-being, companies contribute not only to the health of their workforce but also to increased productivity, job satisfaction, and overall societal well-being.

Government policies play a pivotal role in shaping the health of a society. Policies that support healthcare access, preventive measures, and health promotion contribute to a healthier population. This includes regulations on tobacco and alcohol, support for vaccination programs, and initiatives to address social determinants of health, such as poverty and education disparities. A healthier society requires a commitment to evidence-based policymaking that prioritizes the well-being of all citizens.

In the modern era, technology and innovation offer unprecedented opportunities for improving health outcomes. From telemedicine and health monitoring apps to advanced medical treatments and precision medicine, technological advancements can enhance healthcare accessibility and effectiveness. Integrating technology into healthcare delivery, while ensuring privacy and ethical considerations, contributes to a more efficient and responsive health system.

The health of the planet and the health of its inhabitants are intertwined. A healthier society recognizes the importance of environmental stewardship for current and future well-being. Policies and practices that promote sustainability, reduce pollution, and mitigate the impact of climate change contribute not only to a healthier environment but also to the health of the population. Sustainable practices, such as clean energy initiatives and waste reduction programs, align with the goal of creating a society where both people and the planet thrive.

A roadmap for a healthier society is a dynamic and interconnected framework that addresses the various dimensions of well-being. It involves a collective effort from individuals, communities, governments, and institutions to create an environment that fosters health, equity, and resilience. By prioritizing accessible healthcare, preventive measures, mental health support, holistic education, community engagement, healthy urban planning, workplace well-being, evidence-based policies, technological innovation, and environmental stewardship, societies can pave the way for a healthier and more sustainable future.

This roadmap is not a one-size-fits-all solution but a guide for tailoring interventions to the unique needs and challenges of different communities. As we navigate the complexities of health and well-being, continuous collaboration, innovation, and a commitment to the principles of equity and inclusivity will be key to realizing the vision of a healthier society for generations to come.

CONCLUSION

Empowering Individuals for Lasting Health

Health is a holistic concept that extends beyond the absence of illness to encompass physical, mental, and social well-being. In the pursuit of lasting health, empowerment emerges as a pivotal approach that places individuals at the center of their own well-being. Empowering individuals involves equipping them with the knowledge, skills, and resources needed to make informed decisions about their health and actively participate in their own care. This comprehensive exploration delves into the multifaceted aspects of empowering individuals for lasting health, examining the role of education, self-awareness, preventive care, and community support in fostering a culture of empowerment.

The foundation of empowering individuals for lasting health lies in health education and literacy. An informed individual is better equipped to understand the intricacies of their own body, recognize early signs of potential health issues, and make informed decisions about lifestyle choices. Health education should be a continuous process that starts in schools, providing children and adolescents with the knowledge and skills necessary for making healthy choices. Additionally, adult education and accessible health information resources contribute to raising health literacy levels across diverse populations.

Empowerment in health begins with self-awareness and mindfulness. Individuals need to develop an understanding of their physical and mental states, recognizing the interplay between lifestyle choices and well-being. Practices such as mindfulness meditation, self-reflection, and journaling can enhance self-awareness, helping individuals connect with their thoughts, emotions, and physical sensations. Mindfulness also plays a role in stress reduction, promoting mental health and overall resilience.

Empowering individuals for lasting health involves a shift towards a preventive healthcare mindset. Rather than waiting for symptoms to manifest, individuals are encouraged to engage in proactive measures to prevent illness and maintain well-being. Regular health check-ups, screenings, vaccinations, and lifestyle modifications contribute to early detection of potential health risks and interventions that can prevent the progression of diseases. This preventive approach not only improves individual health outcomes but also reduces the burden on healthcare systems.

Empowerment extends beyond the medical realm to embrace holistic wellness and lifestyle choices. Lifestyle medicine emphasizes the impact of lifestyle factors, including nutrition, physical activity, sleep, and stress management, on overall health. Individuals are empowered to take charge of their well-being by making informed choices in these areas. Integrating principles of holistic wellness into healthcare models encourages a comprehensive approach that addresses the root causes of health issues rather than merely treating symptoms.

A key aspect of empowerment in health is the creation of personalized healthcare plans tailored to individual needs. This involves collaborative decision-making between individuals and healthcare providers, considering factors such as genetics, lifestyle, and personal preferences. Personalized plans may include customized diet and exercise regimens, as well as targeted interventions for managing specific health conditions. By involving individuals in the decision-making process, healthcare becomes more patient-centered and aligned with the unique aspects of each person's life.

Advancements in technology offer a wealth of tools that can empower individuals in managing their health. Mobile apps, wearable devices, and health monitoring technologies provide individuals with real-time data about their physical activity, sleep patterns, and vital signs. These tools not only facilitate self-tracking but also enable individuals to set and achieve health-related goals. Telehealth platforms further empower individuals by providing convenient access to healthcare services, reducing barriers related to time and geography.

Empowering individuals for lasting health involves recognizing the influence of social determinants on well-being. Strong community support and social networks contribute to mental and emotional resilience. Social connections can provide individuals with encouragement, accountability, and a sense of belonging. Community-based programs, support groups, and initiatives that foster social engagement contribute to a culture of health empowerment, creating environments where individuals feel supported in their health journeys.

Financial health is a critical component of overall well-being. Empowering individuals involves addressing barriers to healthcare access related to financial constraints. Policies that ensure affordable healthcare, health insurance coverage, and support for low-income individuals contribute to a more equitable healthcare system. By addressing financial barriers, societies can empower individuals to seek timely and appropriate care, preventing the exacerbation of health issues due to financial constraints.

Empowering individuals for lasting health includes the development of emotional intelligence and resilience. Emotional intelligence involves recognizing and managing one's own emotions as well as understanding and empathizing with others. Building resilience enables individuals to navigate challenges, bounce back from setbacks, and maintain mental well-being in the face of adversity. Emotional intelligence and resilience are essential components of overall health empowerment, supporting individuals in managing stress and maintaining a positive outlook on life.

Public advocacy and health literacy campaigns play a crucial role in fostering a culture of health empowerment. These initiatives aim to raise awareness about health issues, debunk myths, and provide accurate information to the public. Health literacy campaigns, whether through traditional media, social media, or community events, empower individuals to become active participants in their health. By equipping people with knowledge, societies can empower individuals to make informed decisions, ask critical questions, and advocate for their health needs.

Empowering individuals for lasting health is a dynamic and interconnected process that requires a comprehensive and collaborative approach. From health education and preventive care to personalized healthcare plans, technological tools, and community support, the elements of health empowerment are interwoven into the fabric of daily life. As individuals become active

participants in their health journeys, the ripple effects extend to families, communities, and society as a whole.

The shift towards health empowerment requires a commitment from healthcare providers, policymakers, educators, and individuals themselves. It involves breaking down barriers, fostering a culture of collaboration, and recognizing the multifaceted nature of well-being. As societies continue to evolve, the empowerment of individuals in their health will be instrumental in creating resilient, informed, and thriving communities. The journey towards lasting health empowerment is not a destination but an ongoing process of learning, adapting, and embracing the principles of self-determination and well-being.

Real-life Examples of Disease Reversal and Prevention

Disease reversal and prevention are critical aspects of public health, and several real-life examples demonstrate the effectiveness of various interventions and lifestyle changes in achieving these goals. These examples span a range of health conditions and showcase the impact of proactive measures in promoting health and well-being.

1. Cardiovascular Disease: Ornish Program

Dr. Dean Ornish, a renowned cardiologist, developed the Ornish Program for Reversing Heart Disease. This comprehensive lifestyle intervention focuses on a plant-based diet, regular exercise, stress management, and social support. In a landmark study published in the Lancet, participants who adhered to the Ornish Program showed significant regression of coronary atherosclerosis over a one-year period. This approach demonstrated that intensive lifestyle changes could not only prevent but also reverse heart disease.

2. Type 2 Diabetes: Diabetes Prevention Program (DPP)

The Diabetes Prevention Program, a large clinical trial, aimed to prevent the onset of type 2 diabetes in individuals at high risk. The study found that lifestyle interventions, including a balanced diet, regular physical activity, and modest weight loss, reduced the incidence of diabetes

by 58% compared to a control group. This underscores the powerful impact of lifestyle changes in preventing the progression of type 2 diabetes.

3. HIV: Treatment as Prevention (TasP)

In the field of infectious diseases, Treatment as Prevention (TasP) has been a groundbreaking strategy in managing HIV. Antiretroviral therapy (ART) not only helps individuals with HIV live healthier lives but also significantly reduces the risk of transmitting the virus to others. By achieving viral suppression through consistent and effective treatment, individuals can prevent the transmission of HIV to their partners, highlighting the dual benefit of treatment for both personal health and public health.

4. Obesity: The Look AHEAD Study

The Look AHEAD (Action for Health in Diabetes) study focused on individuals with type 2 diabetes and obesity. The study investigated the impact of an intensive lifestyle intervention that included a calorie-controlled diet and increased physical activity. Results showed that participants in the intensive lifestyle intervention group experienced greater weight loss and improvements in cardiovascular risk factors compared to those in the control group. This study emphasizes the role of lifestyle interventions in tackling obesity and its associated health risks.

5. Smoking Cessation: Tobacco Control Policies

Various countries have implemented successful tobacco control policies to prevent and reverse the adverse health effects of smoking. Australia, for example, introduced plain packaging for tobacco products, increased taxes on cigarettes, and implemented aggressive anti-smoking campaigns. Over time, these measures have contributed to a decline in smoking rates and related health benefits, including a reduction in cardiovascular diseases and certain cancers.

6. Malaria: Bed Nets and Antimalarial Drugs

In the realm of infectious diseases, particularly in malaria-endemic regions, the use of bed nets treated with insecticides has proven effective in preventing the spread of the disease. Additionally, antimalarial drugs, when used as preventive measures in high-risk populations, have shown success in reducing the incidence of malaria. These interventions underscore the importance of a multi-faceted approach to prevent and reverse the impact of infectious diseases.

7. Liver Disease: Hepatitis C Treatment Advances

Advances in the treatment of hepatitis C have led to the potential for disease reversal. Direct-acting antiviral drugs have shown high efficacy in curing hepatitis C infection, preventing the progression of liver disease, and even allowing for the reversal of liver damage in some cases. This represents a transformative shift in the management of a chronic viral infection with significant implications for liver health.

8. Alzheimer's Disease: Lifestyle Interventions

While no cure exists for Alzheimer's disease, research suggests that certain lifestyle interventions may help prevent or slow its progression. These interventions include regular physical exercise, a

heart-healthy diet, cognitive stimulation, and social engagement. The FINGER study, conducted in Finland, demonstrated that a multidomain lifestyle intervention could improve or maintain cognitive function in at-risk individuals, providing hope for the potential to impact the trajectory of Alzheimer's disease.

9. Cervical Cancer: HPV Vaccination

The introduction of human papillomavirus (HPV) vaccines has been a significant breakthrough in preventing cervical cancer. HPV vaccination has the potential to eliminate persistent infections with high-risk HPV types, reducing the risk of cervical cancer development. Successful vaccination programs in several countries have contributed to a decline in HPV-related infections and associated cancers.

10. Rheumatoid Arthritis: Early Intervention and Treat-to-Target Strategy

In rheumatoid arthritis, early intervention and a treat-to-target strategy have demonstrated success in preventing disease progression and achieving remission. Aggressive management with disease-modifying antirheumatic drugs (DMARDs) in the early stages of the disease can prevent joint damage and improve long-term outcomes. This approach highlights the importance of early detection and intervention in autoimmune diseases.

These real-life examples underscore the transformative impact of various interventions in preventing and reversing the course of diseases. Whether through lifestyle modifications, targeted treatments, vaccination programs, or public health policies, these successes inspire hope for a future where more diseases can be effectively managed and, in some cases, reversed. The key lies in continued research, innovation, and a commitment to implementing evidence-based strategies that prioritize health promotion and disease prevention.